Bill Phillips
Transformation

Bill Phillips
Transformation

The **Mindset** You Need
The **Body** You Want
The **Life** You Deserve

HAY
HOUSE

For information contact:

T-Media, Inc.
10100 Santa Monica Boulevard
Suite 1300
Los Angeles, CA 90067

FIRST EDITION
ISBN 978-1-4019-1176-8

Printed in the USA

Join Bill Phillips online at transformation.com

Thank you all so much for your help with this project. ~Bill

Paige Dorian • Leigh Rauen • Chris Monck

Chelsea Cordner • Heidi Carignan • Clarissa Lupton • Gail Kingsbury
Suzanne (Mom) Phillips • Rob Cordner • Joe Polish • Stoney Grimes
Marty Goldman • Shane Anderson • Sharen Martin • Chris Winters
Valerie Fontanez • Melissa Sisneros • Penny Ragusano • Carolynn Lovejoy
Spencer Cassler • Debbie Stinson • Katrina Buening • Eric Simpson
Paul Hughes • Chris Rile • Leslie Groft • Stephanie Flynn
Patrick Condren • Joe Pimental • Tyson James • Ami James

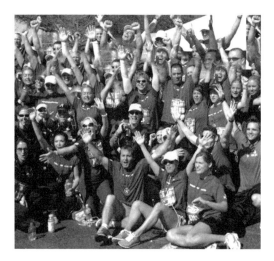

This book is dedicated to the most supportive,
encouraging, authentic and openhearted people
I've ever met: The Transformation Community.
I am forever grateful to all of you. This book
wouldn't be here without your help.

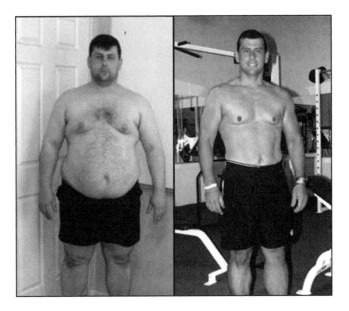

**CHRIS RILE, AGE 34, LAS VEGAS, NEVADA
FATHER AND ELECTRICIAN**

Every night was pizza night. I got up to 325 lbs. I was waiting to die. I'd given up and was just going to bed every night thinking, "I hope it's painless."

I always felt disconnected from the world around me. I used my body weight in some ways to keep me isolated. I was so difficult that my wife left with our son who had just turned two. I remember seeing them drive away and thinking, "That's it. I'm doomed."

I don't know what would have happened if I hadn't joined the transformation. I saw this video of Bill Phillips talking about goals and how to change. That was the catalyst which got me going. For me, the emotional and mental weight is what had to go first.

After 18 weeks I was already halfway there. So I continued on. In 36 weeks I had become over 110 lbs lighter. I started to wake up and see that people, my family, is what's most important. I reached out to my wife Jenn and we started our friendship all over again. After some time, we decided to get back together. Now I've got a second chance to be the father my son has always deserved. Transformation has given me the life I've always wanted.

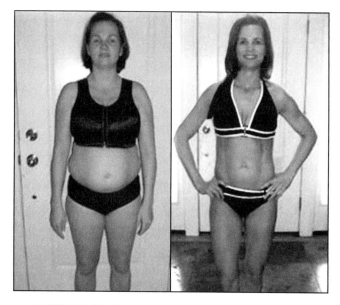

LESLIE GROFT, AGE 35, ENOCH, UTAH
MOTHER OF SIX

Slowly but surely I had gotten away from the healthy person I was back in college. For many of my adult years, I wasn't living consciously. I wasn't exercising at all and I was eating horribly.

My turning point came on New Years Eve, 2008. I was with my husband and we were staying at a beautiful hotel and had planned to go out to celebrate. I just couldn't do it though. I was feeling so much anxiety and depression that I could no longer go out and really participate in life.

A few weeks later I found Bill Phillips at transformation.com and my journey began. My daughter Kylee asked if I was trying to look depressed in my before photo. The answer was absolutely no. That is how I looked and how I felt at that time. The image convinced me that I had to do this and I had to give it all I've got.

After 18 weeks, I couldn't believe how much I'd changed. I reduced my weight by 35 lbs and emotionally I'm so much lighter. Now I can keep up with our six kids throughout the day and still have the energy to exercise. Most important of all, I discovered I can do challenging things. I'm also having fun and participating in life again.

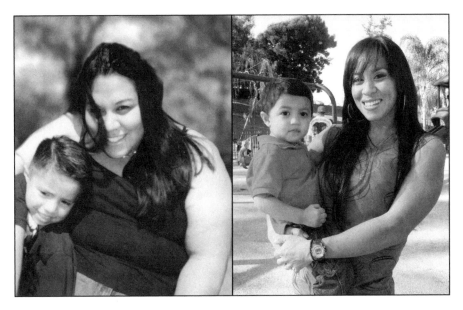

VALERIE FONTANEZ, AGE 30, LOS ANGELES, CALIFORNIA
MOTHER AND GRAPHIC DESIGNER

I was always known as the thick, fat girl. Never in my life was I in good shape. When I was pregnant with my first son I gained even more weight. At my heaviest, I was 260 lbs. I was binge eating just to try to escape the shame and guilt about what I had become. That worked for a few moments but then the negative feelings came back even stronger. I was terrified I wasn't going to be around for my son and husband. That's why I wanted to change. Also, I wanted to do it for myself. I wanted to be healthy.

It's not easy starting out. I had to make a commitment to change each day. Every time I'd see progress in my body or notice I was feeling better about myself, it just gave me that extra push and determination to work harder. I'm now over 100 lbs lighter and I've been able to keep the weight off and sustain my new lifestyle for several years so far.

I believe anybody can do it. If I can change my mental focus and totally rebuild my body then anything's possible in life. I plan to not go back to the old Valerie. This is the new me. And this is how it's going to stay forever.

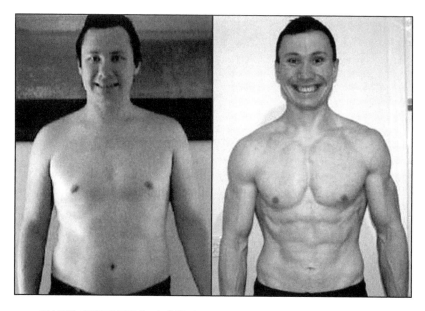

PAUL HUGHES, AGE 35, MELBOURNE, AUSTRALIA
FATHER AND MANAGER

When I first found transformation.com I looked around and saw people who were making incredible changes. Bill Phillips wasn't just teaching fitness but rather how to be healthy and energized from the inside out. People were discovering more of their potential as well.

I dove in and started doing the transformation work. As the weeks went by, I was pleasantly surprised with what I was experiencing. My body was getting leaner and stronger while I also started to feel a renewed sense of purpose. I connected with other healthy and inspired people who were working hard to improve their lives also.

I realized that to some extent, I was living a selfish life, always focused on my job, my fitness, my success. Now I've turned it all around. Today the most important things to me are being the best dad I can be for my two daughters and the best husband for my wife.

I'm also completely committed to making a difference in the lives of others in any way I can. I have an inner happiness and enthusiasm that is greater than before and I share it as often as I can. To me, that's what transformation is all about.

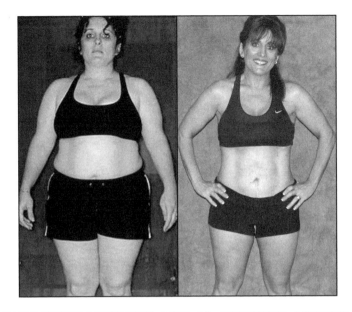

CAROLYNN LOVEJOY, AGE 46, GILBERT, ARIZONA
MOTHER AND SALON OWNER

My life had become very dark. I was always angry, very judgmental. I remember having an anxiety attack at work and I thought, "I just can't do this anymore." I relied on cigarettes and junk food just to get through the day. My kids thought I was going to die and I wondered if they would be better off without me.

I had tried to lose weight many times before. But when I found transformation, Bill asked me to take a different approach. Instead of trying to feel good by losing weight, I was now being taught how to lose weight by feeling good. With the support of people on transformation.com I began to confront my biggest fears and I took a good, honest look at myself. I learned how to process and let go of my anger, how to forgive myself, and even how to love myself.

My body is more than 60 lbs lighter now and I never really had to focus directly on losing weight. When I changed my mind and heart the weight just started coming off. I haven't smoked in over a year. My kids give me hugs and kisses and "I love you's" all the time now.

Today, when I look in the mirror I see a healthy person. I believe in and have respect for myself again.

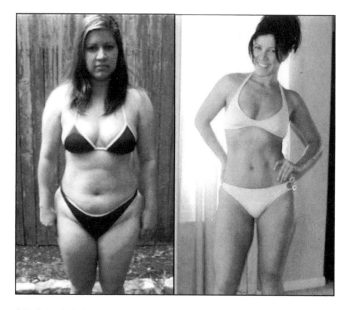

CLARISSA LUPTON, AGE 38, AUSTIN, TEXAS
SUCCESS COACH AT TRANSFORMATION.COM

I had followed Bill's fitness program before and got in good shape, but I lost it all after my baby brother passed away in 2002. I suffered with the most painful grief and depression for so long after that. I gained weight and barely had the energy to get through work and take care of my daughter.

In 2007 I found Bill online and reconnected. He talked to me about transformation and I knew immediately this was something I needed to do. I had never taken the time or knew how to make the inner transformation. The loss of my brother compounded the challenges I had already been struggling with. When you grow up being told that you're a failure and that you'll never amount to anything, it has a way of eating you up inside.

Transformation helped me finally get the healthy body I wanted and more importantly, it allowed me to start living a joyful and fulfilling life.

Now I teach what I've learned to others at transformation.com. Through the community I've made friends all over the world who can relate to my experiences. It's a group of people who are so loving, so supportive and so real.

Now it's your turn.

*"This is the great error of our day, that
physicians separate the soul from the body.
The cure should not be attempted
without the treatment of the whole,
and no attempt should be made
to cure the body without the soul."*

-Plato 427-347 B.C.

Contents

Introduction

Transformation is a process of changing the whole person to become healthier, happier, lighter, more energized and aware. And that's what this book is all about.

Since I wrote Body-*for*-LIFE 11 years ago I've continued to delve deeper into the nature of what true transformation is all about. I poured myself wholeheartedly into the study of the world's great healing traditions from cultures ancient and modern. I became a humble student, open and willing to learn. I was fortunate to get to meet and have lengthy discussions with many mentors whose knowledge in specific aspects of inner change was significantly further ahead of what I knew at the time.

After several years of travel I went to work culling over what I had discovered, identifying key common denominators in all the various teachings and traditions. I then sought to verify and crosscheck this new knowledge through the independent findings of modern science. I was pleasantly surprised to see that an abundance of published, peer-reviewed research studies did in fact exist which confirmed and extended the wisdom I had collected through my travels.

Throughout this past decade, I have put what I learned to work in my own life. My transformation journey has been both humbling and empowering. It wasn't always easy; in fact, there were times when the process became so challenging that I didn't know for sure if I could get through it or not. It was in those difficult times that I transformed the most.

Within this book I share the up close and personal stories of the steps I took to expand my awareness, redirect my mindset, and heal emotional bumps and bruises from the past. I also discovered a spiritual connection I never before knew even existed. All the while, I grew beyond my expertise in athletic performance and fitness, to a new realization of what true health and well-being is all about. As a result, now in my mid-40s, I feel as happy, healthy, fulfilled and enthusiastic as I've ever been. And as I continue to do the work, my life just gets better and better.

For the past few years I've been teaching what I learned to others at seminars, workshops and online at transformation.com. At first I wasn't sure that people would be open and receptive to the depth of these new lessons but as time went on, I discovered a lot of people, from all over the world, who were not only willing to receive what I had to share, but it seemed as though they had been looking for or even anticipating it.

As people began to apply this knowledge and consistently follow through with the action steps, their lives began to change. Yes, their bodies were becoming lighter and stronger, but the real transformation was taking place inside. They began to awaken and more clearly see their true nature, purpose, strengths, as well as potential.

As they continued on, it became more and more obvious that we were no longer just treating symptoms which were showing up in the physical body; we were getting to the root cause of the difficulties within. Inspired by their progress and results, I made the decision to step back up to my writing desk and author this book which brings all of these new lessons to light in one easy-to-read guide.

It's my intention to help as many people as I possibly can and make them aware of the full spectrum of opportunities, which are within their reach, to truly transform their health and life on every level. I also want to let people know that they are closer than they might have ever imagined to being as healthy and happy as they've ever been. I know this through what I've experienced firsthand, and what I've witnessed in the lives of so many others. Consider, for example, the story of Marty Goldman.

A grandfather and small-business owner who lives outside of Chicago, Marty turned to transformation during the most difficult days of his life. He received a phone call on January 1, 2008. It was the most devastating news that any parent could ever hear; his son Tom, an Iraq war hero and father of three, had died. In his shock and grief, Marty had an eerie feeling that if he didn't change his life, he would be the next one to go.

I had met Marty a few weeks earlier at a seminar I was speaking at in Arizona. When I got the news of what happened, I knew immediately what to do. So I got on a plane, flew to Illinois, and went to Marty's home to offer my help. At the time, he weighed over 260 lbs, had little energy, and was well on his way to a heart attack. We talked about his son and family and even though we were just getting to know one another, it felt as if we had been friends for the longest time. Marty realized that his grandchildren were going to need him more than ever now that their father was gone. I told him about some of the people who'd been through the transformation process and how they had recovered their health and renewed their lives. I emphasized—I promised—that he could do it too.

Marty thought about it for a bit and then shared some of his concerns. "I'm getting older, you know. This is what life brings." He continued, "I've tried to lose weight before, change my mindset, and get back on a healthy path but it's never worked for me. How do I know if I try again it'll be any different?" Over the years, I've heard these kinds of words hundreds of times and I've come to recognize they are the kind of perceptions and beliefs that so often interfere with our health and limit our growth in life. I explained to Marty that this time would be different and that the process would be much more than diet and exercise. My approach is based on the concept of holism, which recognizes each person as having an inseparable link between their body, mind, heart and soul. That being the case, we work on all of these areas throughout the transformation process.

I also let Marty know that he was not going to have to do this alone because I would connect him to an unconditionally supportive community, made up of people who had already been through the program as well as others who would be doing the work along with him. I shared with Marty that these people would not let him fail. It was at that point Marty officially made the decision to trans-form for himself and his family in honor of Tom.

Marty says, "I remembered when I first saw my before photo. I never really thought I was fat, I believed I was big. But when I saw that picture, holy cow, I real-ized that I wasn't just fat, I was obese, I was a mess. It was the first time in a long time that I really took a good honest look at myself."

He continues, "I said to myself, 'This is where you're at. You got yourself into this, now it's time to get yourself out of it.' I saw a fat, depressed, unmotivated guy who had no sense of purpose and who had just let himself go. I vowed to never see that version of me again."

That first photo lit a fire within Marty and he became more determined than ever to transform his body and life. And for 18 weeks, he gave his all to each step of the process. The result? He became 71 lbs lighter going from 263 to 192 lbs. His doctor's report showed that he had lowered his cholesterol, blood pressure, and significantly reduced his risk for heart disease. The changes on the inside were just as extraordinary.

"Through the transformation community I've made friends all over the world. I have confidence in myself. I have energy. I'm much happier. Before, I never felt that I really mattered. And now I know I do. I feel like my life has purpose and that I have something valuable to offer others," Marty enthusiastically reports.

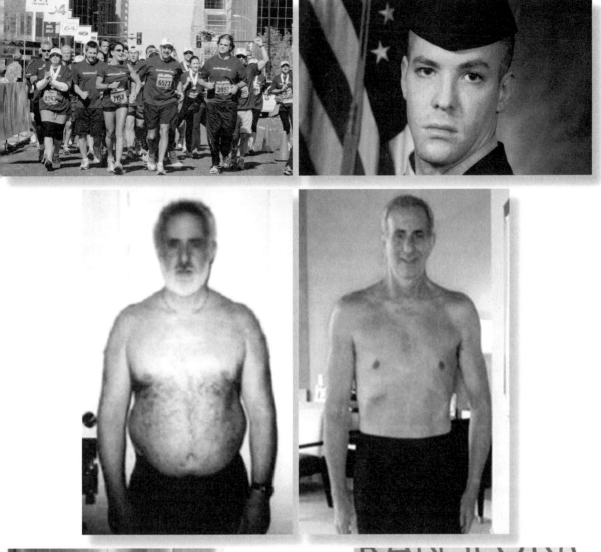

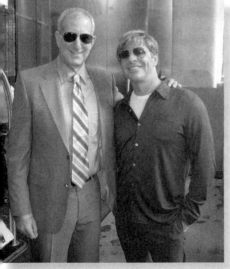

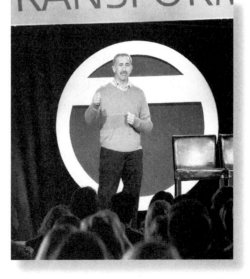

A few months later, Marty and I ran our first marathon together and I could barely keep up. All the while I'm thinking here is this guy who could hardly walk up a flight of stairs when I met him at the beginning of the year and now he's got more energy and endurance than even I do!

After the run, I asked, "Did you ever imagine that you would come this far, this fast?" He looked at me with the biggest smile and said, "Never in a hundred years could I have imagined that my life would be like this. I didn't know it was even possible." But there he is, walking, talking, living, breathing proof that when you make the decision to change and wholeheartedly commit to it, your life will never be the same.

Marty became the very first of our new Transformation Champions and today, over two years later, he weighs right about 192 lbs, he looks 15 years younger than he did before, he's stronger than he's ever been, and his energy is sky high. Now he works full time traveling the country, speaking to groups, and inspiring others to transform their lives too, by sharing what happened in his.

And Marty's not the only one. Already, hundreds of people have applied the transformation steps which I've gathered together and included in this book. Their changes too have been remarkable. Men and women, of all ages, have overcome years of depression to become happier and healthier than they thought they would ever be again.

People who've struggled with addictions to alcohol, cigarettes, drugs and even food, have set themselves free from the chains of their harmful patterns. Many others have become 50, 80, even 100 lbs lighter in less than a year.

All of them have discovered that they had the power to change all along; they just needed direction, support, and the encouragement to tap into it. Now, they're making a difference by sharing what they've learned with others as they continue on, further improving their lives and realizing more and more of their God-given potential. Here in this book, you'll discover all you need to know to follow in their footsteps.

It all begins with a scientifically safe and sound exercise and nutrition plan, designed to help you reduce bodyfat while gaining strength and energy. Transformation then goes beyond the body, integrating a total of 18 action steps which will help you develop greater emotional well-being, mental clarity, peace of mind, as well as a higher level of spiritual awareness and connection. The full initiation process requires 18 weeks. That's not a lot of time compared to how long it's taken to get into the unhealthy situation to begin with.

I invite you to read through the whole book so you can see what the transformation process is all about. Then, I encourage you to come back and focus on one chapter per week. Read, study and contemplate the wealth of knowledge and practical wisdom in each of them. You'll find that each lesson includes practical action steps that help you take what you've learned and put it to work in your own life so you can enjoy the benefits and internalize the information.

Even if you just apply what you'll learn in the first four chapters, you would be well on your way to developing a more positive mindset, as well as a lighter, healthier body. Adding any one of the next 14 assignments will help you lift your results to the next level. The most ambitious way to approach this new transformation program is to complete all of the 18 lessons in just 18 weeks. That's called the 'Transformation Challenge.'

Just like Marty and the many others who are enjoying good results, you don't have to go through it alone. With our support groups at transformation.com you can connect with many enthusiastic people who will assist and encourage you. I'm there as well, helping to guide people along with weekly videos, audios and blogs. I've also designed an online workbook which can help you complete each week's assignment.

Through our live radio show, which airs each week on transformation.com, I answer questions and offer key insight about how to get the most out of each step of the process. You can also sign up online to participate in our official challenge, where those who make the most inspiring changes are rewarded with up to

$50,000 and are invited to share their stories at our local meetings and onstage at our national seminars.

Everything about this program has been designed with one intention: to help *you* succeed. What's more, this plan and path have been proven effective by the men and women who've gone before you. The fact that they've done it really does indicate **you can do it too!**

So now I ask, "Are you ready to begin your very own transformation journey to a healthier, happier life?"

If your answer is "Yes" then please, turn the page and let's begin.

1

The Base and Summit

Colorado has *53 fourteeners*.

"What's a fourteener?" you might ask.

It's a rocky mountain that has an elevation of over 14,000 feet. These are big, beautiful mountains that reach far into Colorado's crystal-clear blue skies.

Each summer, beginning when I was seven years old, my Dad would get the whole family together, including my brother, sister and Mom, and we'd all pile into our little Volkswagen, then make the hour-long drive from Golden, a small town at the base of the foothills where I grew up, to the rugged Continental Divide. This mountain range is home to many of the towering fourteeners. It was there that my family spent a great deal of time when I was growing up. In fact, climbing these mountains is my most vivid childhood memory. By age 12, we had ascended most all of them. Each was a lot of work, up to a 12-mile trek, which could take a full 8 hours.

Looking back today, I realize my Dad knew exactly what he was doing. He was helping me learn, by direct experience, essential skills for a successful

9

and fulfilling life. For example, I learned that before taking on any challenging endeavor, it's vitally important to know both your base (point A) and summit (point B). Once you've clearly defined those points, then and only then is it possible to choose the right path for getting there.

I also learned to never climb alone. It's not safe and the risk of failing to make it to your destination is too high. It is also essential to properly plan and prepare for the climb before you begin. And, once you get started, you have to take it one step at a time and stay focused on the moment you're in.

Another lesson I learned is that there is a high probability that you'll experience adversity, even setbacks, during the climb. For example, the weather changes fast in that part of the country. It can be clear and sunny skies when you begin, but by the time you reach halfway, the sun can disappear behind rolling dark clouds with high-voltage lightening and booming thunder which echoes through the mountains. And then, of course, pouring rain, even snow in early June and late August is not uncommon. It does little good to hold on to the fear that this might invoke. So I learned to feel the fear fast, let it run, and let it go. I also learned to stay close to my climbing group, especially in times of adversity. Any time I'd slip and fall, I'd simply reach out my hand and someone in the group would be there to help lift me back up.

Beyond that, what can I say? It just takes a lot of good old-fashioned hard work to get to the top. There were times when I didn't think I would ever get to the summit; it just seemed too far to go, and my body was doing a remarkably good job of convincing my mind that I had reached my limit. But halfway up the mountain is never a good time to quit. It was then I learned to dig deeper and tap into my heart and soul to find the energy to continue on. Every time I did, I discovered more of my true inner strength.

Standing there on top of the highest mountains in the Rockies, knowing the amount of work, energy, and determination it took to get there, made it all worthwhile. From the summit, the view is always incredible and inspiring.

Through these experiences, I began to learn that setting and achieving challenging goals is a remarkably powerful way to discover your strengths, work on your weaknesses, and build self-esteem.

Today, I'm still climbing mountains. My aspiration of helping to transform the nation from worst to first in terms of health and well-being within my life-time, and perhaps even within 10 years, is Mount Everest to me. In a way, it's a ridiculously challenging goal, and one many people say is impossible. But in my mind and to my understanding and belief, *it is possible*. I feel it and know it. And yet I realize the only way to get there is one step at a time. As I see it, each and every individual health transformation is a step in the right direction and a necessary one to get where we want and need to go. Which brings me to you and your personal transformation journey. My intention is to do everything I can to help you reach the summit of the mountain you decide to climb.

YOUR TRANSFORMATION JOURNEY: GETTING STARTED

For me to help you achieve success in your transformation journey, we both need to know, right up front, two vitally important things:

1) Where you're starting from.

2) Where you're going to.

Without these two key coordinates it would be impossible to measure your progress and success. It also makes it difficult for others to support and help you along the way. But when you are clear about where you are and precisely where you're going, I and others will be able to know and understand what this climb is all about for you and we can help you get there.

Think about it. When you don't know where you're going, how can you tell if you ever get there? You can't. You're going to be lost at the beginning, middle and end. Consider the example of a GPS system in a modern car: In order for it to work, we need to clearly define our present location and where we want to end up.

To me, the meaning of transformation is quite simple and it pertains to just what we're talking about here. It's going from one point to another, or more specifically, one state of being to another.

The iconic symbol of the butterfly communicates this as well as a couple more important points which help us define transformation. Long before the Internet, before books, before most people could even read or write, symbols and allegories were the universal language, conveying concepts directly to the psyche or soul. Today, such archetypes continue to speak to us. And in this case, the metaphor of caterpillar to butterfly connotes three things:

1) Transformation is going from a lower to a higher state of being.

2) It's the ending of something old and the beginning of something new.

3) There's a degree of permanence, of irreversibility to it.

As we move forward, keep these points in mind as they are important differentiators between this process and conventional diets, workout programs and other self-improvement plans which deal merely with exterior issues. Whenever we try to change ourselves from the outside in, it never lasts. We lose weight only to gain it back. Or we might get motivated for a short period of time but it doesn't last. We might temporarily change our habits and patterns through self-restraint, but individual willpower is simply not enough to keep us on the right path for any considerable length of time.

You see, as long as we're still the same inside, at the level of our thoughts, beliefs, patterns, and emotions, we simply haven't undergone true transformation. It's because inward processes always precede external forms and events. And so that's where we begin; we turn our attention inward to take a look at where we are now with this first step of self-appraisal.

Where are you now in regards to your state of being?

That can be a tricky question to answer so let me help point you in the right direction with this following list of self-inquiries and action steps.

HEART AND SOUL

Having looked inward to do some soul-searching, three heartfelt reasons for making the decision to transform my health and life are:

Example:

1) I want to set a healthy example for my kids to follow.

2) I've been taking care of other people, but neglecting myself. Now I'm going to renew my health and energy so I have more to give.

3) I'm tired of being tired and I'm ready to feel energetic, inspired, and confident again!

The deeper and more heartfelt your reasons, the better and more satisfying your results will be. Yes, most all of us want to look a little better, but beneath that, what are the *real* reasons for making the decision to transform? When we identify those, it can really help motivate us to both start and sustain the effort required.

EMOTIONS

In recent days and weeks, the three most predominant inner feelings I have been experiencing are:

Example:

1) Unsettling concern about my weight and heart health; fearful that I might not live my full life.

2) Embarrassed and ashamed about my condition, to the point that I don't get out and do things like I used to.

3) Frustrated because I feel stuck in the situation I'm in.

You may or may not be able to relate with the emotions in this example. Some people come into this program already doing pretty well. For them, the transformation might be making the change from good to *great*. What's important is for you to both identify and then document *your* feelings at the

13

beginning of this process. You can do that with a simple spiral notebook or, as I mentioned earlier, you can fill out the assignments through the online workbook, which you'll find at transformation.com.

MINDSET

Three patterns of thinking or beliefs which may have limited my ability to change in the past are:

Example:

1) Other people can lose weight and become healthier, even happier, but I can't. This is just the way I am.

2) I don't have the time for exercise and eating healthy.

3) It's too late for me, I'm too old.

Now again, this example may or may not be something you can relate to but we all have patterns of thinking and beliefs which may limit our potential, no matter where we are on the path. And there's always a next level; in fact, that higher level seems to always be calling on us to break the barriers of our current condition and reach up for it. Essential to making that leap is continually bringing these kinds of limiting thoughts and beliefs into the light of our conscious awareness so we can see them for what they are: *misperceptions.*

BODY

Three objectively verifiable statements which reflect my physical condition right now are:

Example:

1) My weight first thing in the morning, before I've eaten, is 217 lbs. My mid-section measurement at the widest point is 46 inches.

2) My total cholesterol level is 234 ng/ml. My blood pressure is 142/87 as measured by my doctor.

3) My present physical condition is evident in my before photo.

Notice in the first example, all that's required is a bathroom scale and a tape measure. Both of these can be very helpful in describing your starting point, but I don't recommend that you base your daily or even weekly success on these measurements as we move forward. Once we get started, we'll be focusing much more on evaluating daily progress by whether we've done the work we need to do in order to help our bodies and lives transform from the inside out.

Using a tape measure or scale to check in on your physical results is something I would only recommend doing every two to four weeks. Far too often people rely upon the scale to tell them how they're doing, which is a mistake. You see, your weight each day can fluctuate several pounds based on the amount of water and food your body is holding. Because of this variation, weighing yourself often is not a very accurate way to measure your progress. People who get caught up in this become frustrated and that negatively affects their motivation and confidence.

Trust me, the results will be there in the long run if you simply take it one step at a time and do the work you need to do to get there. You'll learn all about that work as you continue on with the subsequent chapters.

To describe your starting point in even more detail, you can document health indicators such as your total cholesterol level and blood pressure which is something your doctor will be happy to help you do.

And finally, to complete this process of self-evaluation, it's time to take a before photo. To do this, guys simply throw on a pair of shorts, stand face forward with no shirt and have someone snap a quick picture. Alternately, you might be able to set your camera on an automatic timer, stand in front of it and get the snapshot. Gals, you'll want to do the same thing except, of course, wearing shorts and a sports bra or tank top. I know this step isn't one most people look forward to doing, but it is absolutely essential to get it done.

LOOKING FORWARD 18 WEEKS

And now it's time for a really fun part of this assignment. I need you to look forward to a point 18 weeks from now and envision what you want the results of your transformation to be. Again, to help guide you I've got a set of self-inquiries.

HEART AND SOUL

Looking forward, 18 weeks from now, three changes I will have made that show I'm more aligned with what's important to me at a heart and soul level are:

Example:

1) I will be setting a healthy example for my whole family and we'll all be getting healthier together.

2) By making the time to take care of myself, I will have more positive energy and strength to share with others.

3) I'll feel good about myself and my heart will be more joyful which will allow me to participate in life and have more fun with it all.

What I believe you'll discover by going through this process is that your heartfelt *reasons* for making the decision to transform will become a part of your new and improved life. What's more, those changes will make a difference in the lives of others.

EMOTIONS

Looking forward, 18 weeks from now, the three most predominant inner feelings which describe what I'll be experiencing are:

Example:

1) I will be more confident and secure about my overall health and my doctor will report that my total cholesterol and blood pressure are now within the optimal range.

2) I'll feel good about the improvements I've already made and excited about continuing the journey.

3) I'll feel more energized and inspired because I'm moving forward in a positive direction for the first time in a long time.

Very often, the most profound changes people experience by going through this process are in their emotional condition. That's because, more than anything else, we experience life through our feelings. It's not really being out of shape or overweight that bothers us; it's *how we feel* about it. As you'll learn later in this book, positive emotional states like happiness, inspiration, and gratitude contribute to the health of your body.

MINDSET

Three new patterns of thinking or beliefs which expand my ability to make healthy changes for the better will be:

Example:

1) My results will offer proof that I really can make healthy changes in my body and life.

2) I'll show I do have time for exercise and eating right; in fact, on the days I work out, I'll discover I can get more done because I'll have greater clarity and focus.

3) I'll prove it's never too late to make healthy changes physically, mentally, and emotionally!

Make no mistake, when you set your mind in the right direction, your transformation will take off. By mindset I mean your patterns of thinking and beliefs. When those are limited by misperceptions about your true abilities, it always interferes with your efforts to change. The good news is that when you expand and improve your thinking and adopt new, empowering beliefs, you'll enjoy much greater success.

17

BODY

Three objectively verifiable statements which will describe the new and improved condition of my body 18 weeks from now are:

Example:

1) My weight first thing in the morning before I've eaten will be 188 lbs and my mid-section measurement at its widest point is 34 inches.

2) My total cholesterol level will be below 200 ng/ml and my blood pressure will be in the optimal range which is below 120/80.

3) My after photo will show that my body looks much healthier than it did before. There's less bodyfat, firmer muscles, and a youthful posture. You'll see an authentically confident and joyful smile too.

Please note that these statements are your physical health transformation **goals**. It's important to write them in a way that's specific, measurable, and objectively verifiable. Saying, "I want to be in great shape," isn't enough. That's like telling the GPS system in your car that you want to, "Go to some place that's really beautiful." Those descriptions are subjective; they can mean different things to people. Goals are different in that they're objectively verifiable; they look the same to everybody. For example, becoming 30 lbs lighter, as measured by a scale, is clear and absolute.

Goals also have a specific timeline and deadline built in. It's not enough to say, "Someday I want to become 30 lbs lighter." The statement, "Within 18 weeks, I will become 30 lbs lighter," is a specific, objectively verifiable goal. Most people aren't used to deciding precisely what it is they want to achieve so this might not come naturally to some. It is, however, a vitally important part of this process and it's one that holds significant power. In fact, research findings of the world's leading experts in the field of setting and achieving goals cite that those who set the most concrete and specific objectives are the ones who are most likely to experience the best results.

Once you've reached this point, be sure to read your goals often; I read mine every morning and every night to help me stay focused on achieving them and to determine how to invest my time in the day ahead.

Envisioning the condition of your new, transformed self, which your goal statements describe, is also beneficial. Some of the successful people I've worked with over the years make 10-20 minutes available each day to picture how their leaner, stronger, more energetic body will look and perform. There seems to be significant power in doing this and it's something I highly recommend. It's also very helpful to share your goals with others who will be a part of your support structure during the transformation process. The more clearly they understand your specific objectives, the more they'll be able to help you successfully reach them. Got it? Good!

CONCLUSION

By the time you complete this assignment and become clear about where you are in the present, and where you want to be in the future, you will have taken a big step in the right direction. You'll become remarkably clear, perhaps more than ever before, about what changes you want and need to make in order to feel good about your progress and life. You may also be pleasantly surprised at how inspired and enthusiastic you become about getting where you've decided to go. The rest of this book is about helping you get there. It's something I know you can do. By the time you reach your summit, you'll know it too. I promise.

19

2

Exercise Rx

Most everyone knows that exercise is good for you, yet few understand *how good* it really is. Yes, working out helps burn calories, enhance weight loss and strengthen muscles. But did you know that exercise has been scientifically shown to make us more intelligent, happier and more successful? It's true!

When I first started developing exercise programs for people 25 years ago, there was little if any recognition from the mainstream medical community that there was any real benefit to it. In fact, some health care professionals would often warn against it, propagating myths like endurance training is bad for your heart and weight lifting would make you 'muscle-bound' and limit physical performance.

Fast forward to today—*so much is changing*. Physician and Vice President of the American College of Sports Medicine, Robert Sallis M.D., explains it this way: "Exercise can be used like a vaccine to prevent disease and a medication to treat it. If there were a drug with the same benefits as working out, it would instantly be the standard of care." Yes, if the health-enhancing effects of exercise could be put in a pill, it would be the best-selling pharmaceutical there ever was, as well as the safest and most effective.

A new call to action takes it a step further. **Exercise is Medicine** is the name of the program organized by a group of doctors and health care professionals which calls on physicians to assess and review each patient's physical activity levels at every visit. Their mission, which I endorse and support 100%, is to make exercise a standard part of disease prevention and treatment in the United States. The group believes that doctors should prescribe exercise to their patients just as they would a life-saving medicine. Ultimately they see this leading to a paradigm shift in modern medicine, one that will lead to tremendous overall improvement in the public's well-being and substantial long-term reductions in health care costs. Their recommendations support a growing body of evidence that working out does much more than burn calories and strengthen muscles.

A study published in the *Journal of the American Medical Association* (2005) revealed that consistent exercise can double survival rates of breast cancer patients. Researchers followed 3,000 women being treated for the disease and found that for those with hormone-responsive tumors, walking the equivalent of 3-5 hours per week at a moderate pace, cut the risk of dying from the disease in half compared to the sedentary women in the study.

These findings confirm and extend previous scientific studies which show that exercise significantly strengthens the body's immune system. Harvard Medical School reports that more than 60 studies in recent years make clear that women who exercise regularly can expect a 30% reduction in their chances of developing breast cancer to begin with.

Researchers at Duke University studied people suffering from depression for 4 months and found that 60% of those who exercised for 30 minutes, 3 times a week, overcame the condition without using antidepressants which is about the same percentage rate as those who use medication only in their treatment of depression. And of course, exercise is not only a mood brightener, it produces dozens of other positive effects which antidepressant drugs simply do not.

There is now considerable evidence derived from hundreds of studies, with thousands of subjects, which prove that exercise is remarkably effective in relieving symptoms of depression and anxiety. The best results were shown to occur in vigorous (intense) exercise performed consistently. And the benefits continue as long as someone continues to work out.

Exercise not only helps resolve symptoms of depression and anxiety, but it also enhances self-esteem, produces more restful sleep, and helps people recover more quickly from adversity and better cope with social stress.

I'm not basing these claims on a single study. They are supported by what's called a 'meta-analysis' which is a report that essentially combines the findings of most, if not all, of the available research on this topic in the English language. The overall positive patterns of these studies make it remarkably clear that exercise plays an important role in promoting sound mental health and emotional well-being. It works for men and women, adolescents, adults, and senior citizens too.

A study by the California Department of Education, involving 954,000 students grades 5, 7 and 9, showed that the most healthy kids (the ones who scored highest on fitness tests and had lower levels of bodyfat) did twice as well on aptitude exams in reading and mathematics compared to the least fit kids. Harvard professor, John Ratey, M.D., writes, in his latest book *Spark: The Revolutionary New Science of Exercise and the Brain*, that more physical fitness for students is a cure for not only unhealthy weight gain, but also the kids' academic performance.

Additional research shows that consistent exercise protects us from the common cold, flu, and bacterial infections by elevating the body's production and circulation of immune cells. Exercise has even been shown to strengthen people's response to the influenza vaccine, making it more effective at keeping deadly viruses at bay. In addition, exercise boosts blood flow to the brain which helps it receive more oxygen and nutrients and it increases the energy of brain waves that are responsible for quick thinking, focus, creativity, and problem solving.

German researchers recently compared a group of athletes to others who were healthy non-smokers but not regular exercisers. The athletes had significantly less degradation in the strands of DNA at the tips of chromosomes called 'telomeres.'

When telomeres begin to shorten, cells can no longer divide and they become inactive, a process associated with aging, cancer, and heart disease. The German study was published in the November 2009 edition of the *Journal of The American Heart Association* where it concluded physical activity has a profound anti-aging effect at the cellular level.

Studies at Tufts University in Boston have demonstrated that even at age 92, moderate-resistance exercise, performed 3 times a week for 8 weeks, increases muscle strength by an average of 174%. This translates into a 48% increase in mobility and a significant reduction in fall risk.

Another study, published in the journal *Neurology*, looked at 3,298 folks with an approximate average age of 70 years. Over a 9-year span, those who participated regularly in vigorous exercise (tennis, jogging, biking, swimming, weight lifting) were discovered to be 63% less likely to suffer a stroke compared with inactive senior citizens.

Exercise has been shown to both prevent and treat osteoporosis, help manage diabetes, reduce the risk of addiction relapse, slow premature aging of the skin, promote healthier digestion, reduce aches and pains, contribute to optimism and a positive mindset. What all this information points to is that exercise is not a silver bullet—*it's platinum.*

24

THE PRICE OF INACTIVITY

The fact that such remarkable benefits come from simply adding a few hours of exercise to our weekly schedules begins to make clear how devastating the effects of inactivity actually are. You see, what exercise does is simply reverse the damage done by living a sedentary life. If exercise is a vaccine, as Dr. Sallis puts it, inactivity is akin to a deadly virus.

Medical experts now say *inactivity poses as great a health risk as smoking*. Let's pause here for a moment to process that. Okay, what that means is if parents let their kids play video games and sit at the computer all day, it's akin to handing them a pack of cigarettes. Yes or no... would you do that to your kids? And what about yourself?

Please realize that every week you don't get up and move for a few hours (walking, weight lifting, jogging) takes you another step closer to heart disease, diabetes, hypertension, cancer, depression, arthritis, and osteoporosis. Again, I'm asking you to pause, take a deep breath and consider what this means in your life and the lives of those you know and care about.

This next statistic is both stunning and sad: According to the *Archives of Internal Medicine*, more than 80 million U.S. adults don't do any voluntary exercise at all. And we wonder why America, this great nation with an abundance of resources, technology, and scientific know-how, is dead last on the list of the health of modern countries.

Making people aware of the reality of this situation can literally save lives. It's true! It's also true that if we can get this message out and get people moving, we can transform the nation from worst to first in health and fitness. We start by setting a positive example for our families and friends. We can ask them to participate with us—invite a buddy to the gym, take the kids to a park and kick off a friendly game of soccer, shoot baskets, go swimming or race in the backyard. Do something, anything, that gets the blood and oxygen pumping, lights up the brain and works the muscles!

On the one hand it seems too simple; how could working out or walking help change the nation? Yet when we look at the bigger picture and consider all the scientific evidence that we've reviewed so far, the impact of your leading by example and helping to spread the message makes a very real difference in the future of our society.

Add to this the devastating financial consequences: Last year it cost our country over $147 billion to take care of citizens who didn't take care of themselves. How can there be true health care or financial reform without getting every man, woman and child that can participate in a few hours of weekly physical activity to do so? I think the only way that's possible is to individually and collectively get up, get moving, exercise, be active and bring as many people with us as we possibly can!

THE RIGHT DOSAGE

Oftentimes people mistakenly believe that to enjoy the benefits of exercise they would need to dedicate a significant portion of their day to it. Television weight-loss reality shows that feature people working out 6 hours a day contribute to this widespread misunderstanding. The scientific fact is that significant psychological and physical health benefits begin to occur with as little as 30 minutes of walking, 3 days a week. This is something virtually everyone can do so they don't miss out on this vitally important aspect of the transformation program.

If you're just starting out with an exercise program or are coming back to it after considerable time off, be sure to first check with your doctor (he or she will very likely give you the thumbs up and even congratulate you on your decision) and then simply start out gradually with a couple hours of exercise per week. It really can be as simple as walking or jogging for about a half hour every other day. You could also use indoor aerobic equipment like a treadmill, stair-climber or stationary bike.

Swimming, yoga, tennis, bicycling, martial arts, hiking... those are all good forms of exercise too. Adding in some weight lifting each week offers tremendous benefits as well.

After you've been consistently exercising for a month you can increase the 'dosage' for even more benefits by adding another hour of exercise a week or by increasing the intensity of your workouts. For example, if you've been regularly jogging at a 12-minute per mile pace, you can aim for an 11-minute pace and when you get comfortable with that, take it to 10 minutes per mile.

With strength training, we can increase intensity by adding more weight to our lifts; for example, if we've been doing 3 sets of 10 repetitions on the shoulder press with 20-lb dumbbells, we can increase it to 25 lbs and the next month aim for 30 lbs. This is called 'progressive-resistance training' and it's the foundation of every effective strength-training program. What I teach athletes and weekend warriors is that if you want to build muscle, you've got to get stronger and stronger. This style of training also produces tremendous benefits in terms of building bone mass and reinforcing tendon and ligament strength.

Vigorous exercise also helps increase the metabolic rate which is how many calories the body uses up to keep going all day long. Scientific studies have shown that after a good workout, our body burns more fat throughout the day. This is why simply keeping track of the calories burned during exercise is not really an accurate way to measure energy expenditure.

All these recommendations are within the U.S. Department of Health and Human Services (HHS) Physical-Activity Guidelines for Americans. Having worked with HHS as a part of a task force assigned to develop solutions for childhood obesity in particular, I've gained considerable respect and appreciation for the credibility and validity of their work. The HHS guidelines, published in 2008, are the result of thousands of hours of analysis of the available scientific literature (hundreds and hundreds of studies) on physical activity and health. I wholeheartedly endorse and support their findings which follow:

U.S. DEPT. OF HEALTH AND HUMAN SERVICES EXERCISE GUIDELINES FOR ADULTS

- All adults should avoid inactivity. Some physical activity is better than none, and adults who participate in any amount of exercise are going to gain some health benefits.
- For substantial health benefits, adults should do at least 150 minutes (2 and a half hours) a week of moderate-intensity, or 75 minutes (1 hour and 15 minutes) a week of vigorous-intensity aerobic exercise, or an equivalent combination of moderate and vigorous-intensity aerobics. Aerobic activity should be performed in episodes of at least 10 minutes, and preferably, it should be spread throughout the week.
- For additional and more extensive health benefits, adults should increase their aerobic exercise to 300 minutes (5 hours) a week of moderate-intensity, or 150 minutes (2 and a half hours) a week of vigorous-intensity aerobic exercise, or a combination of moderate and vigorous-intensity activity.
- Adults should also do muscle-strengthening exercises that are moderate or high-intensity and involve all major muscle groups on 2 or more days a week, as these activities provide additional health benefits.

MORE EXERCISE INSIGHT

The HHS recommendations accurately reflect that the greater the effort level, the less time is needed to produce positive effects. With a more moderate-intensity level, the duration of the exercise session needs to be longer to get results. This supports what I've been teaching for well over a decade which is, when it comes to working out, quality (intensity) matters significantly more than quantity (duration).

A study in the journal *Metabolism* showed just how effective High-Intensity Interval Training (HIIT) actually is for decreasing bodyfat levels. In this 20-week study, one group performed HIIT on a stationary bike for about 30 minutes per workout while another group performed a more traditional, slow-paced aerobic routine for 45 minutes. In this study, the HIIT workout involved starting with 5 minutes of pedaling at a very moderate pace to warm up. Then it evolved into performing short, intense bursts of sprinting (pedaling as fast as they could for about 60 seconds), followed by a couple minutes of very slow pedaling to lower the heart rate back down to 120-130 beats per minute. This sprint-rest cycle was repeated 10-15 times.

At the conclusion of this study, the HIIT group lost over three times as much bodyfat as those following the traditional aerobic workout. This happened in spite of the fact that the endurance group expended twice as many calories during their workout. The researchers discovered that for every calorie expended during HIIT, there was a ninefold loss of subcutaneous bodyfat as compared to the endurance trainers.

Again, this indicates that we can't measure the fat-burning effects of exercise by simply looking at the calories-expended number on high-tech aerobic equipment. What's happening is a significant amount of stored bodyfat is being burned in the hours after the workout. In fact, this study showed that there was an increase in the lipase enzyme activity and beta-oxidation (fat burning) in test subjects who did the HIIT program. This metabolic effect was not seen in those doing moderate-aerobics.

Those familiar with the Body-*for*-LIFE workout, which I developed back in 1999, will recognize that the 3 weekly 20-minute, high-intensity workouts combined with 30-40 minutes of weight training, 3 days a week, performed on alternate days, fits right in with these important HHS recommendations. The Body-*for*-LIFE exercise method is a remarkably effective routine which has worked well for hundreds of thousands of people. It is not, of course, the only efficacious approach to training. There are many 'right ways' to work out. What I suggest is to pick one which fits your schedule and is also convenient as well as practical for you. Then, just get started and never stop!

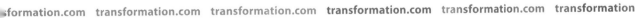

It's vitally important that we plan our exercise sessions in advance. They should be incorporated into your daily schedule and adhered to just as if they were an appointment at the doctor's office. You can plan a week in advance or the night before your day begins. You'll want to know where you're going to work out, what time of day, and which exercises you're going to do. Just a small amount of planning can make a big difference in terms of compliance.

You can work out at home or a health club/gym or a combination of both. When I'm traveling, I enjoy stopping into 24-Hour Fitness health clubs and Bally's fitness centers. When I'm not on the road I enjoy exercising at home and as often as possible, I get outdoors to do my aerobic training. For home workouts all you need is a set of basic free weights and an exercise bench which you can purchase at a sporting goods store, or even Walmart.

I have included detailed video demonstrations of the most effective free-weight exercises on transformation.com so you can see the proper form, tempo, and safety tips. You'll also find specific training programs from people who've enjoyed tremendous success in their transformation process. I share examples from people who've become over 100 lbs lighter while gaining energy and healing depression. There are examples of men who've burned off 30 lbs of bodyfat while putting on 10 solid lbs of muscle. You will also see exercise examples from women who've made remarkably healthy changes. Finding someone who's made the kind of changes you'd like to make and following in their footsteps can be a very effective approach. The fact that they've done it will allow you to see and believe that you really can do it too.

At transformation.com you can also receive support and encouragement from people who've been through the process and who enjoy helping others by answering their questions and offering insight. You can join one of our online support groups to connect with others from around the country, even around the world, who are at your fitness level. I'll teach you more about the tremendous benefits of participating in a support group like this in Chapter 4.

MY EXERCISE ROUTINE

Now that I'm over 40, I am less concerned about building big, 'ripped' muscles and more focused on the overall health benefits as well as the preventative medicine aspects of exercise. With that in mind, I do 2-3 weight-training workouts a week, each session lasting about 40 minutes. In each exercise session I'll work all the major muscle groups of the body or I'll split it up and do upper body on Monday and Friday, lower body on Wednesday. I've posted some videos showing the exact workouts I do online at transformation.com.

For cardiovascular fitness and weight management I perform 20-30 minutes of intense aerobic exercise or HIIT, 2-3 days a week. I do this on days when I don't weight train. Whenever the weather allows I get outside and do a few miles of interval training where I walk a couple minutes, jog a couple minutes, then sprint for 30-60 seconds. Then I start the walk-jog-sprint cycle over again. I do this 4-6 times per workout. It's remarkably effective and very challenging! When I can't get outside to train, I take the same approach on a stair-climber or stationary bike indoors.

I prefer to work out first thing in the morning, but depending on my work and travel schedule, I sometimes end up training in the afternoon or evening. The important thing is not so much when you exercise but rather making sure you get it done.

ACTION STEP

Based on the scientific evidence presented in this chapter, three specific exercise benefits that I am now holding the intention of personally experiencing are:

Example:

1) Healthy and sustainable weight management.

2) Increased energy and brightened mood.

3) Actively practicing preventative medicine to lower the likelihood that I would ever suffer from chronic conditions such as diabetes, depression, cancer, and heart disease.

The amount of time I will make available for exercise each week throughout this 18-week transformation journey is:

Example:

I will exercise for a total of 3 hours weekly. I'm going to do 3 intense, 20-minute aerobic workouts each week for a total of 1 hour. On alternating days, 3 times per week, I will do 40 minutes of strength training for a total of 2 hours.

Someone I can share my exercise plan with at the beginning of each week so he or she can help keep me accountable to my goals and intentions is:

Example:

A friend, family member, personal trainer or accountability partner from the online transformation community.

Someone I can offer support, encouragement and friendly accountability to throughout this 18-week program is:

Example:

A friend, family member, someone in the transformation community.

CONCLUSION

Exercise is good medicine. It's a healthy prescription which can help you improve the condition of your mind and body. And it's something that can benefit everyone: men, women and children alike. It will help you form a solid foundation of well-being and give you the mental energy and clarity to complete the challenging assignments and action steps ahead. The sooner you begin, the sooner you will enjoy the many benefits.

3

Right Nutrition

Thank goodness there's always opportunity wherever we find a problem because when it comes to the way we eat in America today, we've got a big one.

Our country has become the least healthy modern nation in the world; over 160 million Americans now suffer from overweight and obesity which is, to a significant extent, caused by unhealthy eating habits. It's literally an epidemic which has already reached nearly 70 percent of our entire population. The number of overweight American children has quadrupled in just a generation while the number of overweight adults has doubled. Statistics show that one out of every two babies born today will develop diabetes in their lifetime if things don't change.

What's more, other modern nations around the world are following our example. At a recent meeting of the International Congress on Obesity (a coalition of more than 2,500 experts and health officials), chairman Paul Zimmet, M.D., Ph.D. concluded: "This insidious, creeping pandemic of obesity is now engulfing the entire world. It's as big a threat as global warming."

And Dr. Philip James, British Chairman of the International Obesity Task Force, has gone on record stating, "We're dealing with a problem that, it is already accepted, is going to overwhelm every medical system in the world."

This big problem is destroying human health and well-being at an unacceptable rate. It's one that's impacted each and every one of our lives—if not you personally, someone you know and love.

OVERFED AND UNDERNOURISHED

As a society, we're stuffed but starving. We're getting too much quantity and not enough quality. The typical American menu is simply too high in calories and too low in nutrients. I call this calorie toxicity, nutrient deficiency. Because the body needs essential nutrients to thrive it will keep telling us to eat more food so it can try to meet its needs. This can lead to constantly craving but yet never satisfying our body's true nutritional requirements.

Nutrient deficiencies lead to immune system suppression and subsequently illness and disease. Everything from muscle and bone loss to rapidly aging skin and headaches, to irritability, anxiety, and depression have been scientifically linked to the inadequate nutrition millions of people experience. Thank goodness, the opposite is also true! And that means, when you learn how to eat the right way, your mind will become more alive, your immune system stronger, and you will feel younger, healthier and happier.

What I find is the more understanding and clarity people have about how to eat right, the better and faster they can both let go of unhealthy body weight and increase their energy, vitality and well-being. So that's what we'll focus on in this chapter.

DIETS DON'T WORK

The fact is, restrictive diets don't work. They can't work. Not now, not ever. They're not just ineffective, they're potentially dangerous and most always a dead-end street. Dieting is like going underwater and holding your breath.

Eventually you have to come to the surface, and when you do, you gasp for air and inhale all you can. It's the same way with trying to go without eating. No matter how hard you try, eventually you'll give in, and you'll eat, sometimes even binge, gain weight and lose self-esteem.

Another reason that restrictive diets don't work is because, by and large, the objective is to merely cut calories, with little or no regard for repairing nutrient deficiency. The result is that the body may temporarily become smaller and weigh less but overall health and energy are not improved.

So dieting isn't the answer; eating right is. I've been studying, researching and writing about this for over 20 years now and I can tell you, it's really not that complicated. Once you learn what you need to know about this, you'll always know it and you'll be able to apply it, when you choose, for the rest of your life.

THE 7 ESSENTIAL NUTRIENTS

It all starts with foods that provide the high-quality, essential nutrition your body needs. The technical term for these foods is 'nutrient rich and calorie sparse.' That's the opposite of what we find in most highly processed foods, junk food and fast food which are high in calories and low in nutrients.

To eat right, we need to include in our meals healthy sources of the 7 nutrients which I consider *essential* to great health: quality protein, good carbs (carbohydrates), essential fats, vitamins, minerals, phytonutrients and water.

Unfortunately, many people today aren't getting enough of these nutrients or the right balance of them. Scientific research shows there's widespread deficiency in vitamins, minerals and essential fats especially, which as we've already discussed, causes poor health. When we bring things back into balance and start feeding the body the nutrients it needs, you'll begin to enjoy the benefits within a matter of days. Let's take a closer look at these 7 essential nutrients now.

PROTEIN

Protein is a *very* important nutrient; in fact, the word itself originates from the Greek word meaning 'of prime importance.' Along with carbohydrates, protein is a 'macronutrient,' meaning that the body needs relatively large amounts of it. Vitamins and minerals, which are needed in only small quantities, are called 'micronutrients.' Unlike fat and carbs, the body does not store extra protein so it has no reservoir to draw on when it needs a new supply. Good sources of quality protein include: chicken, turkey, beef, fish, eggs, soy, milk and protein powders derived from it, especially whey protein.

These foods offer complete proteins which contain all nine of the essential amino acids: histidine, isoleucine, leucine, lysine, methionine, phenylalanine, threonine, tryptophan, and valine. (By the way, knowing the essential amino acids by name plus 4 bucks, will get you a cup of coffee at Starbucks.) The reason these amino acids are 'essential' is because your body can't make them on its own, so they must be provided through the foods we eat.

The amino acids derived from quality proteins are the building blocks of every cell in the body. Muscle, blood, skin, hair, nails, even cartilage, are mostly made of protein. The body also uses protein to make enzymes, hormones, neurotransmitters, and antibodies which support the immune system.

Scientific studies also show that protein helps stabilize blood sugar levels when it's consumed with carbs which contributes to a sort of 'time-released' energy as opposed to spikes up and down. Whey protein in particular has been shown to help stimulate the release of two appetite-suppressant hormones: cholecystokinin (cck) and glucagon-peptide-1 (glp-1). Studies have demonstrated that adding whey protein to a midday snack or beverage provides stable energy and can help control food intake at the next meal. Protein also has the highest 'thermic effect' of any food. This means our metabolism gets a boost when we eat protein and as a result we burn more calories.

36

CARBOHYDRATES

Carbohydrates, like protein, are essential to good health. They are first and foremost a source of immediate energy for all of your body's 75 trillion cells. Carbohydrates also cause the release of insulin, a powerful hormone needed to help amino acids and other nutrients enter cells, which is very important of course. In that way, carbohydrates and protein work together, which is one of the many reasons I include both in every meal.

Eating some protein with carbs helps slow the release of glucose (metabolized from carbohydrates) which in turn keeps insulin levels from going too high. This is especially important for Type II diabetics who need stable blood sugar levels.

In recent years, there has been a great deal of discussion and debate, among diet doctors in particular, about the eminent evils of eating carbohydrates. And although I agree that we over-consume carbohydrates here in America, particularly in the form of refined sugar, that does not mean all carbs are bad for us.

Scientific studies, including several from the Harvard School of Public Health, show a connection between eating whole-grain sources of carbs and improved health. In a study of more than 160,000 people whose health and dietary habits were followed for up to 18 years, those who had at least 2 servings of whole grains a day were 30% less likely to have Type II diabetes compared to those who ate mostly processed sources of carbohydrates.

Eating whole instead of refined grains substantially lowers total cholesterol, triglycerides, and insulin levels. Each of these changes reduces the risk of cardiovascular disease. In a Harvard-based Nurses' Health Study, women who ate 2-3 servings of whole-grain products (mostly bread and breakfast cereals) each day were 30% less likely to have a heart attack or die of heart disease over a 10-year period.

37

Researchers in Australia studying 106 overweight adults put 55 of them on a very low-carb plan and they had another group of 51 adults follow a restricted-calorie, moderately high-carb plan. After a year, weight loss in both groups was about the same, 30 lbs. However, the researchers also evaluated the emotional well-being and mood of the people in both groups. The low-carb group reported especially high levels of anger, depression and confusion after a year on the Atkins-like diet; whereas, the higher-carb group actually improved their emotional well-being and reported that they were very often in a good mood. Researchers suggested a link to better serotonin synthesis with the higher-carb group while those eating less carbohydrates developed a deficiency of this feel-good neurotransmitter.

Sugar is a 'crummy carb' which produces unstable energy levels throughout the day. It's also addictive. Once you get hooked, it takes a significant effort to break free. The 'withdrawal' period, which can last anywhere from a few days to a few weeks, can be difficult to go through, but it's always worth it. Soft drinks, candy, and cookies typically contain a lot of sugar and eating too much of them leads to overweight and obesity, Type II diabetes, and increased risk of heart disease. Suffice it to say, we want to avoid sugar as much as possible.

The good news is, it's relatively easy to incorporate healthy carbs into our daily nutrition plan. Quality sources include: brown rice, potatoes, oatmeal, yams, barley, apples, berries, oranges, grapefruit, bananas, whole-grain pasta and breads.

ESSENTIAL FATS

That's right, *essential* fats. Not unhealthy saturated or trans fats. We need to keep our consumption of those to a minimum. Essential fats are the good, healthy ones. They're called essential because the body can't make them on its own, but yet they are required for many metabolic processes. Therefore, they must be supplied in food or supplements.

Essential fatty acids facilitate the production of hormone-like substances which regulate blood pressure, immune response, and inflammation (in response to injury, infection or stress).

These essential fats are called Omega-6 (linoleic acid) and Omega-3 (alpha-linolenic acid). We tend to get enough Omega-6s through the foods we eat but very often don't get optimal levels of Omega-3s. Perhaps the best sources of Omega-3 fatty acids are cold-water fish such as salmon, tuna, herring, flounder, halibut, swordfish and mackerel. Oils from these fish contain a couple particularly potent forms of Omega-3s called DHA and EPA. There is extensive evidence from a large number of scientific studies which indicates that optimal intake of DHA and EPA reduces risk of heart attack, stroke, depression and arthritis.

Plant sources of Omega-3s such as flaxseed oil, do not contain EPA and DHA. The Center of Science in the Public Interest reports that, "The Omega-3s the FDA considers helpful (EPA and DHA) are not found in plants such as flaxseed." It's possible that the body can make EPA and DHA from the Omega-3s in flaxseed oil but many experts, including the FDA, recommend fish oil sources over plant sources.

There's been some concern that eating too much cold-water fish can lead to unhealthy levels of heavy metals, like mercury, in the body. However, researchers from the Harvard School of Public Health reported in the *Journal of the American Medical Association* that the benefits of eating fish tend to outweigh the potential risks. The World Health Organization publishes acceptable standards regarding contaminates in fish oil; the most stringent current standard is the International Fish Oil Standard (IFOS). Fish oils that typically make this highest grade are those that have virtually no measurable levels of contaminates. In another report, wild salmon was shown to have no mercury while swordfish, tuna and lobster contained some, albeit still a pretty small amount. Salmon is one of my favorites so this works well for me.

Scientific studies are continuing to demonstrate the healthful effects of Omega-3s on body and mind. For example, a study published in the journal *Nutritional Neuroscience* reports a strong potential for fish oils to be utilized as a natural antidepressant. Omega-3s have healing properties when it comes to brain health. In fact, 8% of the brain is composed of EPA and DHA. In a six-month study comparing EPA to a placebo it was found that the people receiving extra amounts of this essential nutrient experienced an increase of gray and white matter in the brain. Omega-3s are important structural components of brain cell membranes as well as the retina of the eye. DHA helps the production of phospholipids of the brain's gray matter suggesting they are important to central nervous function and the availability of neurotransmitters.

The *British Journal of Psychiatry* reported that people who are deficient in Omega-3s tend to have higher rates of attention deficit and are more prone to fitful, even violent behavior. This study followed a group of young adults in detention for disobedience issues. When they were given foods or supplements with richer Omega-3 fatty acid content they were found to have increased attention span and reduced violent behavior. In yet another study it was shown that increasing kids' Omega-3 fatty-acid intake helped them overcome learning difficulties and perform better in the classroom. In adults, research shows that Omega-3 supplementation improves memory, mood and self-management (emotional stability, discipline, thoughtfulness).

Guidelines issued by a workshop on the Essentiality of and Recommended Dietary Intakes (RDI) for Omega-6 and Omega-3 fatty acids, sponsored by the National Institutes of Health (NIH), recommend that people consume at least 2% of their total daily calories as Omega-3 fats. To meet this recommendation, a person consuming 2,000 calories per day should eat sufficient Omega-3-rich foods to provide at least 4 grams of Omega-3 fatty acids. This goal can be easily met by adding just two foods to your daily nutrition plan:

40

flaxseed and wild-caught salmon. A tablespoon of flaxseed oil contains 8 grams of Omega-3 fats, while a 4-ounce piece of salmon contains 1.5 grams of Omega-3 fats. There's research evidence showing that two servings of non-fried fish per week—especially salmon, tuna and halibut—can be enough to significantly increase the level of Omega-3 fatty acids in your blood (including the level of both EPA and DHA).

VITAMINS AND MINERALS

Vitamins and minerals are also essential nutrients because our body needs them to function properly, but it can't make its own supply. So each day, we need to eat foods that are naturally rich with these micronutrients, or those which have been fortified with them. For an 'insurance policy' many experts recommend a daily vitamin and mineral supplement too.

Vitamins and minerals contribute to good health, well-being, muscle growth and energy production by regulating the metabolism and assisting biochemical processes in the body. If you don't get enough of these essential micronutrients you'll experience deficiency symptoms, which include muscle weakness, slow fat loss, connective tissue deterioration, frequent colds and infections due to suppression of the immune system, to name just a few.

Vitamins are either fat soluble or water soluble, depending on whether fat or water-based molecules transport the vitamins through the bloodstream. Fat-soluble vitamins include A, D, E and K. Because these vitamins have an affinity for fat, they can be stored in both adipose (fat) tissue and in the liver, so we don't have to consume them each and every day. The water-soluble ones include all of the B vitamins and C; they aren't stored in the body for more than a few hours, so daily intake is a must.

Minerals are *in*organic in nature, meaning they are not produced by plants or animals. They can, however, be found in food sources, for example, iron in red meat, calcium in milk and potassium in bananas. Minerals are also extremely important for your body to work right. They are essential for nerve cell communication, flexing muscles, fluid balance and energy production. Many minerals also serve as building blocks for body tissues, such as calcium and phosphorus for bones.

Minerals are referred to as either bulk or trace depending on the amount needed by the body. Bulk minerals include calcium, magnesium, potassium and sodium. Trace minerals, on the other hand, may be required in quantities as little as a few micrograms (that's just one-thousandth of a milligram). These include minerals such as chromium, copper, iodine and selenium.

In our daily nutrition plan, we'll want to include good sources of vitamins and minerals in the form of fruits and vegetables, such as apples, oranges, tomatoes, bananas, berries, broccoli and spinach. Also, quality protein and healthy carbs often provide rich sources of essential micronutrients.

PHYTONUTRIENTS (SUNLIGHT NUTRITION)

We're all powered by sunlight. It is the source of energy and life on earth. Sunlight sustains our environment, producing heat and ultraviolet rays which form what we call visible light. Human beings and animals cannot directly transform sunlight energy into fuel for our bodies. We need a mediator to assist in the process, and this is where plant life comes in. Leaves of a plant are like solar panels in that they absorb sunlight and synthesize it (photosynthesis), then store it. When we eat the plants in the form of fruits and vegetables our body does something pretty spectacular: it retrieves the stored sunlight from the plant, thereby releasing and converting the solar energy (in particular the hydrogen ions) to fuel our bodies and minds.

Consider the saying, ***you are what you eat***, not in a literal sense, but rather in reference to the energetic qualities or vibrancy of food. When we look at it that way, we can see how highly processed foods, which have never seen the light of day, are no replacement for natural food sources which carry the energy of the sun. Fresh, natural foods have a high vibrational frequency like light itself. Synthetic foods have a slower, lower frequency and when that's all we eat, we tend to become that way ourselves. Depression, apathy and fatigue have a slow wave pattern whereas health, happiness and vitality have a much more rapid vibe. It's also important to note that sunlight is not just energy, it's information and intelligence-rich energy. This kind of light is also called consciousness and fresh fruits and vegetables are carriers of this.

Some nutrients are especially rich with light. These are called phytonutrients. They're not yet officially classified as essential nutrients according to the FDA as are vitamins and minerals but, from what the science is showing, I believe they should, and eventually will be. The fact is, phytonutrients are necessary for optimal health and they must be supplied by the foods you eat because your body can't manufacture them on its own. From my perspective, that's the definition of what an essential nutrient is.

Phytonutrients are the living sparkles of golden light that contribute to the remarkable health benefits of consuming ample amounts of fruits and vegetables. Now of course plant foods are also good for us because their fiber helps with good digestion; they're rich sources of vitamins and minerals too. No wonder more and more scientific studies are coming to the conclusion that the more fruits and vegetables we eat, the longer and healthier we'll live.

Research at Harvard's School of Public Health reveals that for each daily serving of fruits and vegetables a person eats, they lower, by 4%, their risk of heart disease. Another study shows that for every serving of fruits and vegetables we eat each day, our life expectancy increases by two years. Want to live 10 years longer? Eat five servings of fresh fruit and vegetables every day, this study concludes. The National Institutes of Health reports that when we eat multiple servings of fruits and vegetables we decrease our risk of developing numerous forms of cancer (lung, mouth, stomach, colon, breast, pancreas and bladder). In addition, we can lower our risk of stroke and diabetes.

Scientific studies also show that the phytonutrients in fruits and vegetables work as powerful antioxidants in the body which protect cells against oxidative damage and degradation caused at the microcellular level from normal processes in the body.

Carotenoids, flavonoids, polyphenols, and saponins are all types of phytonutrients which provide antioxidant effects. Green tea is also rich with phytonutrients (polyphenols).

Green tea has also been shown to have significant antioxidant effects which may reduce the risk of cardiovascular disease, dental cavities, kidney stones and certain forms of cancer while improving bone density and cognitive processes. One very interesting study shows that the active phytonutrient or polyphenol in green tea (called EGCG) may have considerable healing effects on brain cells, contributing to what doctors call 'neurorescue' or 'neurorestoration.'

A British university study showed that fat oxidation rates are 17% higher after people drink green tea and their total energy expenditure (calories burned) becomes significantly higher as well. The findings go on to suggest that drinking green tea can help fat burning during moderately intense exercise and also improve insulin sensitivity and glucose tolerance.

Anthocyanins are another especially potent form of phytonutrient. They're found in plants which contain red, purple and bluish colors such as apples, grapes, eggplant, wild blueberries, pomegranates, blackberries, cherries and raspberries. Resveratrol, the phytonutrient thought to be responsible for the protective health qualities of red wine, and acai (ah-sigh-ee) from the palm tree which is of the same name, are also anthocyanins.

Lately, acai has been widely promoted as a 'miracle' weight-loss nutrient and while that may not be completely accurate (well, it's not accurate at all actually), acai, like other phytonutrients which act as antioxidants, does indeed seem to help protect the body from premature aging.

44

Anthocyanins are so good at absorbing and storing sunlight, they're even being utilized in solar panels which generate clean energy and electricity with the potential to power entire cities.

Not a phytonutrient, but definitely a sunlight-dependent one is vitamin D. Our bodies make more vitamin D when the sun reaches and warms our skin. Over the past decade, vitamin D deficiency has escalated to the point where most American adults are deficient in this essential vitamin. Another Harvard School of Public Health study suggests that vitamin D deficiency may also be linked to heart disease as well as osteoporosis and a weakened immune system. Researchers looked at the vitamin D levels of healthy men and checked in on them for 10 years. Their research revealed an alarming statistic: The men who were deficient in vitamin D were twice as likely to have a heart attack compared to those whose vitamin D levels were within the optimal range. Other scientists found that vitamin D plays a role in controlling blood pressure and preventing artery damage.

The vilification of ultraviolet light in recent years has given rise to widespread heliophobia (fear of the sun) which in turn has caused many people to stay out of the sun altogether or only go out completely covered with sunscreens. This is a very new phenomenon obviously, as the sun has been revered and worshiped for thousands of years as a source of life itself which, in the physical universe, as I've already pointed out, it very much is. Experts in the matter cite that 10-20 minutes a day of direct sunlight exposure can help resolve vitamin D deficiency. In addition, extra supplementation of vitamin D is often recommended.

Wonderfully nutrient-rich sources of phytonutrients include: apples, bananas, cantaloupe, grapes, grapefruit, oranges, peaches, pears, pineapple, plums, strawberries, watermelons, asparagus, artichokes, bean sprouts, beets, brussel sprouts, cauliflower, green beans, green and red peppers, lettuce, tomatoes, broccoli, and carrots.

WATER

Absolutely essential to good health is consuming ample amounts of water. Water covers approximately 70 percent of the earth's surface and makes up over 70 percent of our bodies as well. All living things rely on water to thrive, you and I included. It helps produce energy, detoxify the kidneys, regulate body temperature, build new cells and lubricate joints, among thousands of other functions.

We naturally lose water every minute of every day, just through breathing. During the summer months, water losses are greater because body perspiration, which is used to cool our systems, evaporates faster in a hot environment. Caffeinated and alcoholic beverages are diuretics—they cause you to lose even more body water.

Unfortunately, most Americans, research shows, don't drink nearly enough water. Consequently, many people are walking around in a chronic state of dehydration, which is not good to say the least. Water losses of one percent of your total body weight can impair functioning both mentally and physically. Losses of four percent can cause headaches, loss of energy, muscle weakness and irritability. Losses of seven percent can be fatal. Oftentimes, when our bodies need water the sense of thirst is interpreted by our awareness as hunger and that can lead to overeating. So to control the appetite, drink water.

Tap, bottled, distilled or filtered... as long as it's clean, it will get the job done. Moderately active people can stay well hydrated by consuming about an ounce of water for each two pounds of body weight. For example, I weigh 188 pounds so the right amount for me is about 94 ounces a day (188 divided by 2 equals 94). For me that comes out to six 16-ounce bottles of water a day. Endurance athletes who exercise for long periods of time in warm environments may need considerably more. Just remember when it comes to water, drink up and often, to your health!

INTENTION, CONSCIOUSNESS AND FOOD

A recent study offers scientific evidence that there may indeed be a factual basis for what many of us have known for so long... Mom's homemade chicken soup, prepared with love and care, has curative effects. In this study, published in the *Journal of Science and Healing* titled, "Effects of Intentionally Enhanced Chocolate on Mood," individuals were assigned to different groups and asked to record their feelings of well-being each day by using a standard test called the 'Profile of Mood States.'

Each person in the study consumed a half-ounce of dark chocolate twice a day at prescribed times. Some of the chocolate had been prepared with the intention that people who ate the chocolate would experience an enhanced sense of energy, vigor and well-being, and some of the chocolate had not. The study was 'double blind' which means that neither the test subjects nor those doing the hands-on research were aware of which chocolate had and hadn't been treated with intention.

At the end of the study, conducted at the Institute of Noetic Sciences (noetic means the effects of mind or consciousness), the data was processed and the confidential information about which group had been using the placebo was revealed. To a significant degree, those who received the food which was subject to positive intention reported decreased fatigue and increased vigor. The scientists concluded that indeed, the mood-elevating properties of chocolate can be enhanced with positive intention.

The study's lead investigator, Dr. Dean Radin, is a pioneer in the research of the mind's effect on matter. He's been a mentor of mine for the last seven years as well. Dr. Radin explains, "Focused human intention is one of the most powerful forces on earth." He should know, he's worked for decades to understand this phenomenon, conducting extensive research at Princeton and Stanford Research Institute International. Dr. Radin estimates that there are at least 1,000 published studies on some form of intention, including those done by the U.S. military, the Max Planck Institute, Princeton, Harvard and Duke universities.

What this research suggests is that it does matter whether our meals are manufactured by soulless machines, or if they're made in the home kitchen or the local family-owned café, with care and good feelings. It also seems to validate that blessing a meal before we dig in can perhaps help purify or alter the energetic nature of food. Keep in mind that intention, like prayer and blessings, is about the positive energy you feel while you're saying the words, and not necessarily from the words themselves.

As you might surmise, I pause, breathe deeply, and bring to mind and heart a loving, bright, healthy intention while I have my dinner in front of me each evening.

ORGANIC, RAW FOODS, VEGETARIANISM

In recent years, we've seen an increasing interest in natural and plant-based eating plans. Vegetarians, for example, eat fruits, vegetables, cereal grains, nuts, seeds and legumes, but no meat. A lacto-vegetarian plan includes dairy products; an ovo-vegetarian plan includes eggs but not dairy products; and a lacto-ovo-vegetarian eats both eggs and dairy products, but again, not meat. A vegan approach excludes all animal products such as dairy, eggs, and sometimes even honey.

Vegetarianism is oftentimes a part of a person's spiritual path and belief system. There is a theory that the trauma animals experience when bred for commercial meat production is carried in the beef, chicken, and fish. Since science is beginning to substantiate that intention is carried into our bodies from the foods we eat, it is plausible that there could be some transfer of the animals' pain. This is oftentimes a key factor in a person's decision to become a vegetarian. I appreciate and respect those who make that choice.

I think that most anyone who really understands what goes on in the meat-producing industry would want to eliminate or at least minimize the amount of food they consume from those sources. I personally choose wild salmon (as opposed to boring), free-range chicken and eggs, and grass-fed beef only. They cost a little more but I really feel like it's worth it. This is, however, more a matter of personal preference than scientific fact.

Organic foods are also becoming more popular, especially amongst those who are more health conscious. These foods have been grown in environments free of synthetic chemicals including pesticides and growth-promoting hormones. Of course, throughout the vast majority of human history, agriculture could be described as 'organic.' It's really just been within the last few generations that unnatural and potentially unhealthy methods have been employed.

The organic-food industry is very well regulated and the USDA's Organic Seal of Approval is a reliable indicator that a food product has been made by a certified producer. Australia, Japan, Germany, France and the European Union also have credible organic certification standards overseen by the government. Keep in mind though, the word 'organic' can be put on just about any product; it's a valuable catchword in today's consumer market, but it does not guarantee the product is legitimately organic. I've seen the word organic on the label of some very high-fat, unhealthy and processed foods so please be cautious and realize that organic doesn't necessarily mean *healthy* on product labels.

Another trend in nutrition is eating foods raw or at least not cooked at a temperature above 116 degrees. The concept is that foods are more nutritious when they're raw or barely cooked and that they retain enzymes which assist in digestion and absorption of the food. While it's certainly valid that fresh, natural fruits are wonderfully nutritious in their whole, uncooked form, for many vegetables cooking makes their phytonutrients easier to absorb by the body, such as the beta-carotene in carrots. It also may not be critical that foods contain all their original enzymes because the body uses its own to digest and assimilate the food you eat. And so again, following a raw-food plan is a matter of personal preference and philosophy rather than one based on a preponderance of science.

A 'macrobiotic' approach is another eating style that's centered around natural, unprocessed food. Followers of the macrobiotic plan believe that food quality affects health, energy and well-being which, of course, it absolutely does. It emphasizes eating light portions of natural and mostly unprocessed foods including fish and seafood, seeds and nuts, fruits and vegetables. And for some, it also includes milk and yogurt. Macrobiotic daily menus change with the seasons to anticipate a person's energetic and nutritional needs at different times of the year.

When I'm working with people following a vegetarian, raw-food or macrobiotic approach to nutrition, I always emphasize the importance of adequate protein intake. For vegans, both soy and bean-sprout protein powders are available at natural grocery and health-food stores and can be used to make nutrition shakes which help meet the body's protein needs.

Scientific studies suggest that people who follow these kinds of eating styles may be more likely to experience vitamin B12 deficiencies and suffer anemia, but that's typically not something that proper supplementation couldn't resolve. One report, published in the journal *Mechanisms of Aging and Development*, discussed evidence that vegetarians may not live longer than others due to glycation reactions in the body. Glycation is essentially a toxic binding of glucose to the body's proteins which decreases their functions. Yet adequate carnosine supplementation may help avoid that condition. Alternate studies show that people who follow vegetarian eating styles have less heart disease and do indeed live longer. But of course, that's true with any clean and healthy approach to nutrition.

50

MEAL FREQUENCY AND CALORIE MANAGEMENT

I've already mentioned that restrictive diets are not typically sustainable or even healthy. Yet it's vitally important that we keep our calorie intake within a healthy range. If you're trying to lose bodyfat you'll need to consume less total calories than your body burns each day; that requires your body to tap into stored fat to meet its daily energy needs. If you're already in good condition, or when you reach your goal weight, you can eat a little more but still it's important to consume only the amount of calories that your body needs; otherwise you'll start putting the bodyfat back on.

Something I've certainly learned through personal experience is that I need to work with my body, not against it, when it comes to controlling calories. We've got to keep ourselves satiated (satisfied, not starving). And one of the best ways to keep cravings at bay is to eat more often throughout the day, up to six times. When we do this, the body is energized, nourished and satisfied. We also feel lighter, more aware and more energetic as opposed to being weighed down by big meals for breakfast, lunch and dinner.

A scientific study reported in the *European Journal of Clinical Nutrition* cites that people who ate six times a day had a faster resting metabolic rate than those who ate just three meals daily. Your metabolic rate is the pace at which your body burns calories all day and night. This study showed eating smaller meals frequently throughout the day allows people to burn fat more efficiently. Researchers at Georgia State University arrived at the same conclusion. They found that folks who ate just three meals a day had, on average, a higher percentage of bodyfat than those who ate six times per day.

Another study published recently in *The New England Journal of Medicine* showed that in as little as *two weeks*, people who ate frequent, portion-controlled meals as opposed to three large meals (containing the same total amount of food) reduced their 'bad' cholesterol levels by nearly 15%, lowered their cortisol (the stress hormone that contributes to belly fat and premature aging) levels by more than 17% and diminished insulin levels by almost 28%. Another study, this one published in the *International Journal of Obesity and Related Metabolic Disorders*, found that when people eat frequent meals throughout the day it helps control their appetite. A study published in the *American Journal of Clinical Nutrition* reported that people are most successful at losing fat and keeping it off when they eat numerous meals throughout the day.

Another way eating six small, nutritious meals a day helps you reduce bodyfat is by allowing you to maintain muscle mass. Remember, muscle not only helps the body look good but also makes it more metabolically active. Muscle burns calories even when it's just sitting there. Fat does not. In fact, for every pound of muscle you gain you'll burn another 50 calories a day. People who put on 10 pounds of muscle will therefore burn 500 calories more per day. This equals an additional 4-5 pounds of fat burned off every 30 days.

PROTEIN AND CARBS WITH EVERY MEAL

Now that we've talked about the essential nutrients and the benefits of eating more frequently, it's important to understand how to put the right combinations of food together. What I recommend is that every time you eat, you combine protein and carbs. Again, this is backed up by solid science.

For example, a study published in the *Journal of Nutrition* showed that balancing protein and carbs stabilizes blood sugar and insulin levels which led to a decrease in bodyfat, lowered cholesterol and a reduced risk of Type II diabetes. In another study reported last year in the journal *Physiology and Behavior*, a team of Swiss researchers reported that by balancing protein and carbs in each meal, you can benefit not only your body but also your mind. Balanced eaters experienced better overall cognitive performance compared to test subjects who ate meals that were not balanced.

The *European Journal of Clinical Nutrition* published a report that eating a balance of protein, carbs, and essential fats in each meal resulted in greater feelings of energy and lower levels of fatigue. They determined that balanced meals promote stable energy and greater endurance. In the journal *Medicine and Science in Sports and Exercise* researchers reported that for test subjects who exercise, consuming a post-workout meal or nutrition shake with both protein and carbs resulted in improved mood, enhanced feelings of strength, and greater confidence.

Scientists have also shown that people who eat a balance of protein and carbs have better digestion and absorption of nutrients as well as an increased "thermic effect" (fat-burning effect) from each meal. On top of all that, studies show that meals balanced in protein, carbs, and essential fats provide a safe and healthy way to manage the appetite. I've discovered the same thing which is why I eat meals that contain a balance of protein and carbs and I suggest that you do too.

DIABETIC CONSIDERATIONS

Diabetes is a condition in which a person's body has abnormally high glucose (blood sugar) levels either because the body doesn't produce enough insulin or because the body's cells don't properly respond to insulin that is produced. Insulin is a powerful hormone, produced in the pancreas, which helps shuttle glucose into cells where it's used for energy. When the body's cells cannot properly absorb glucose, blood sugar levels become significantly elevated (hyperglycemia) and this can lead to vascular disease, heart attack, stroke, blindness and other complications.

Type I diabetes is most often a congenital condition where natural insulin secretion isn't adequate to maintain good health. Insulin injections are required to manage blood sugar levels each day, throughout life, for those who have this type of diabetes.

53

Another form of the disease affects millions of American adults and children today and is primarily caused by lifestyle decisions including what we eat and our activity levels. This is called Type II diabetes and here, the body does naturally produce adequate levels of insulin, but cell-receptor sites don't recognize or respond to it due to attenuation or down-regulation. This can happen when we eat a lot of processed carbohydrates and sugars, year after year. When we do this, insulin receptors on cells just get hammered by high-circulating levels of insulin, which are released in excess whenever we eat big amounts of highly processed carbs. Unfortunately, with millions of kids and adults consuming so many sugar-packed sodas and junk foods day after day, the rates of Type II diabetes are skyrocketing. Untreated or improperly managed diabetes is fatal.

Medication in pill form can often assist the absorption of blood sugar into cells, but it's essential for anyone facing Type II diabetes to take control of the way they eat, eliminating sugar and processed carbs. Combining a portion of protein and carbs in each meal, and eating smaller, frequent meals throughout the day can help Type II diabetics manage their blood sugar levels and protect their health. When I'm setting up a nutrition program for someone with this condition I'll often recommend only whole-grain carbs for the first three (of six) meals during the day and only vegetables for carbs during the afternoon and evening meals. The amount of carbohydrates they eat each day would be less, perhaps 30% of total calories during a day, compared to about 50% for non-diabetics with my plan. Each person should talk to their physician about what the right approach is for them of course.

The good news is, Type II diabetes can be so well managed with proper nutrition and consistent exercise that it doesn't have to interfere with or shorten a person's life. In fact, I've worked with many Type II diabetics who've turned their adversity into an opportunity to lose weight, become fit and completely transform their health. Now their example inspires others to do the same.

THE ADVANTAGE OF NUTRITION SHAKES

Weight-loss pills which are hyped in television, magazine and Internet ads are akin to fool's gold. Their marketing claims look good, but when it comes right down to it, they have very little value. And that's not all. The FDA has already taken action to ban some diet pills because of their negative effects on health. Fortunately, there's a healthier solution.

Harvard Medical School researcher Dr. George Blackburn led a 10-year study which evaluated the benefits of nutrition shakes on long-term weight management. He followed two groups of men and women (a total of 539 folks) from 1992-2002. The first group followed the typical American pattern of eating and the second replaced two of their daily meals with a calorie-compact nutrition shake. At the end of the 10-year study there was a remarkable difference in the body weight of men and women from these groups. Those who continued to use two nutrition shakes a day were, on average, 33 lbs lighter than those who did not use nutrition shakes. Dr. Blackburn concludes, "This is a scientific, safe approach to weight-control therapy," and goes on to add, "This study proves that yes, we can avoid gaining weight. This epidemic doesn't have to overtake us."

Another study, reported by the National Institutes of Health (NIH) in April of 2009, evaluated 5,145 men and women who successfully lost weight and were able to keep it off. This NIH report revealed that there were three key factors to sustainability: 1) Consistent exercise of 2-4 hours a week; 2) Regularly participating in support groups; and 3) Consuming two meal replacements (nutrition shakes and/or bars) per day. These NIH findings show us precisely what we need to do to sustain healthy weight loss. All three of these key factors are incorporated and recommended as a part of this transformation process. This NIH report is unbiased, objective and has been reviewed and determined valid by doctors and researchers not involved in the study.

Another study, this one conducted at Creighton University and published in the journal *Nutrition & Metabolism* (2008), evaluated the effects of a high-protein nutrition shake (fullstrength.com) which is also balanced with a moderate amount of carbohydrates and fortified with vitamins and minerals. Researchers asked those participating in the study to do a weight-lifting workout 3 times a week, for a total of 10 weeks. At the end of the study, the nutrition shake users gained more muscle, lost more fat and significantly improved their cholesterol levels compared to the group of strength trainers who did not use nutrition shakes.

Nutrition shakes, used as meal replacements or snacks between meals, are effective not because of any especially potent or miraculous effect, but rather because of the simple fact that they help us bring our calorie consumption down while lifting our nutrient intake up. When we accomplish those two things, the body does the rest and we become stronger, healthier, more energetic and lighter. Nutrition shakes are also convenient and cost effective.

I started teaching people about the benefits of utilizing nutrition shakes back in 1990 when I had the wonderful opportunity to work with a pioneer in the field, a brilliant doctor named Scott Connelly. He developed an excellent product called MET-Rx based on extensive research and also what he had learned from helping hospitalized patients, many recovering from surgery, regain their strength and health. I had the opportunity to help get the message out about the product for a few years. It was a lot of fun, very rewarding, and I learned so much about nutrition and health. I remain very grateful to Dr. Connelly to this day.

From there, I acquired a small company named EAS from a couple of smart, young guys in northern California and I introduced my first performance-nutrition shake (obviously inspired by what I learned from Dr. Scott Connelly) called Myoplex under my new brand. Over a million athletes have enjoyed the benefits of that product since I introduced it in 1996, and even though I sold my ownership of that company over a decade ago, I still recommend their products to bodybuilders, football players, and Olympic athletes.

Today, my interests have evolved—I'm not so much interested in big muscle building and sports performance but rather holistic health, good energy and weight management. So a few years ago I went back to the lab with a friend and leading expert in the science of high-tech food design and formulation, and I came up with a new product called Right Light. It's fortified with all the important vitamins and minerals, as well as a full serving of quality protein, which is balanced with a smaller but healthy amount of good carbs. It also contains one of the most powerful phytonutrients we know of, EGCG (from green tea extract), as well as probiotics and enzymes, which improve nutrient uptake and digestion.

Right Light is very low in calories, only 130 per shake. It's also sugar-free, fat-free, lactose-free, and contains no gluten or aspartame (an artificial sweetener that may not be good for long-term health).

I just recently completed another upgrade of the Right Light formula where I added extra amounts of the amino acids glutamine (muscle and immune system support) and tyrosine (for improved mental focus), and we also added in a new and improved flavor profile for both chocolate and vanilla shakes. It's available in ready-to-drink single-servings as well as packets of powder which are blended with water before serving. You can find Right Light in health-food stores and some fitness centers. Proceeds from Right Light sales have been donated to charities and other philanthropic causes. (You can find more information at eatingright.com/RightLight)

The important thing when it comes to nutrition shakes is that you find a product which tastes good to you, that you can pick up for a fair price, and most important of all, that agrees with your body and makes you feel good. There are a lot of good quality products out there today which you can find at health-food and grocery stores.

PUTTING IT ALL TOGETHER

Now I'm going to walk you through an ideal day of good nutrition in my life. What you'll see is that I keep it pretty simple. As I mentioned, my focus is not so much on physical strength and power like it was back when I was in my 20s and early 30s; today I eat with the intention of enjoying the very best possible overall health and well-being. A part of that is keeping my weight within a healthy range which, I've discovered, is a little more challenging now that I'm closer to 50 than 40. I don't take my physical condition to extremes anymore, like getting my bodyfat down to 5-7%. Moderation and balance are remarkably appealing to me these days.

The effects of good nutrition on cognitive performance and neuro-health have become a very keen interest for me, and you'll see that reflected in the way I eat. Today, it seems like I can conceptualize, create, discern, retain and synthesize information as well or better than at any other time in my life which is encouraging. I believe that incorporating 'neuro-nutrients' into my daily meals as well as consistently staying active and exercising will continue to work for me, far into the future. I also make a very conscious effort to stay up-to-date on how nutrition can significantly lower my risk of developing ailments such as heart disease, cancer, Type II diabetes and autoimmune conditions. I apply what I continue to learn to my daily nutrition plan as well.

You'll notice I have something to eat six times a day. That doesn't mean I'm sitting down for a meal each of those times. My breakfasts and lunches are really quick—less than 10 minutes to prepare the food and eat. And my nutrition shake midmeals take even less time than that. I make more time for dinner and often meet friends at my favorite cafés. It's really not that hard to eat out and stick with the plan as long as you know what to order. For me that's simple because I'm always looking for a lean source of protein, some healthy carbs, and steamed vegetables or a salad.

58

When my objective is to reduce bodyfat I eat about 10 calories per day for each pound of body weight. For maintenance, I multiply by 12. And for gaining solid weight (not that I need any help with that) it works to consume a number of calories that equals your body weight times 15. At my weight of around 188 pounds, the amount of calories per day for reducing bodyfat for me is right about 1,880.

Of that amount, I get about 30% (560) of those calories from good sources of protein (fish, low-fat cottage cheese, protein shakes); about 50% (940) from healthy carbs (fresh fruit, steamed vegetables, whole-grain sources); and about 20% (376) from fat (mostly Omega-6s and Omega-3s). There are 4 calories in every gram of protein and carbohydrate which means I'm aiming for about 140 grams of protein each day and 235 grams of carbohydrate. There's 9 calories per gram of fat which means I need to consume less than 40 grams of fat per day. If I were aiming for a higher or lower daily calorie intake, I would still eat six times a day, but I would change the portion sizes of my whole food meals accordingly.

An example of a typical meal is my favorite dinner: grilled salmon, brown rice and steamed spinach. How I determine the right amount to eat is by using what I call the 'portion rule.' For example, I pick an amount of salmon which is about the size of the palm of my hand; that's a proper portion of protein for me. For brown rice (carbs) and spinach (vegetables), I have an amount that's about equal to the size of my closed hand; again, that's a proper portion size for me. We can take the same type of approach with fruit; selecting an orange or apple that's about the size of your closed hand for example.

The portion rule works really well for me and many others because it helps customize the amount of food that's right for us. Palm sizes vary quite a bit but generally, men have a 35% bigger palm and closed hand than women and therefore require around 35% bigger portions of protein and carbohydrates as well as total calories.

A number of the studies I talked about in this chapter mention 'servings' of fruits and vegetables. They're referring to an FDA food pyramid standard. What you might want to remember is that a portion (closed-hand sized) of vegetables like steamed broccoli or spinach for example, is about equal to two FDA servings. With fruit, a portion is about equal to the FDA serving. In my daily nutrition example you'll see I have two pieces of fruit and a healthy portion of steamed spinach and that equals around four FDA servings. I aim for 3-5 servings of healthy fruits and vegetables each day as I described above. Here's how my ideal, daily nutrition plan looks:

8:00 AM—**Breakfast**: Oatmeal with a handful of blueberries and a little skim milk; 4 egg whites and 2 whole eggs, scrambled; 1 slice whole-grain bread, toasted; 16 oz water.

10:00 AM—**Midmeal**: Right Light nutrition shake, apple, and a SOL Light Energy Shot.™ (SOL is a phytonutrient supplement—eatingright.com/SOL)

12:30 PM—**Lunch**: Turkey sandwich on whole-grain bread with lettuce, tomato, mustard, pickles and low-fat cheese; 16 oz water.

3:30 PM—**Midmeal**: Nutrition bar, orange, SOL, 16 oz water.

7:00 PM—**Dinner**: Grilled salmon, brown rice, steamed spinach with 1 tablespoon flaxseed oil blended in; 16 oz water.

10:00 PM—**Dessert**: Nutrition Milkshake mixed in a blender with 4 oz soy milk, one packet vanilla Right Light (powder), and 4 oz Haagen-Dazs frozen yogurt, vanilla.

I also have two more 16 oz bottles of water (Fiji is my favorite) between meals which brings me to a total of about 96 ounces for the day.

This eating pattern I described above is one I aim to stick with six days a week, but on one day of the week I give myself a little more leeway. I used to take it as a 'free day.' It's not a 'cheat day' but rather a day you can feel free to eat however much or little you want.

Today, that tends to be more like a 'free meal' where I might go out to my favorite Italian café or steakhouse for a bit of a feast with friends or family. I can pretty easily get away with this two nights a week and when I'm designing nutrition programs for people I'm working with, this is generally my recommendation as well. It makes the plan more practical, enjoyable, and sustainable.

There's actually a metabolic advantage to having a free day or a couple of 'free meals,' as well as a psychological one. Studies actually have shown that occasionally consuming higher calorie meals can boost the metabolic rate by as much as 10%, well into the following day. In terms of mental well-being, enjoying your favorite foods, regardless of calorie content, once in a while, keeps the program from being overly restrictive, redundant and boring.

I highly recommend planning your daily nutrition ahead of time; I do it the night before so when the day starts, I know what I'm going to eat, when, where and why. Some people have good results planning the entire week at a time and even preparing meals in advance, then refrigerating or freezing them in individual plastic containers. This can really help compliance, convenience, and it is also very economical.

Now I need to ask you a favor: Please don't be too hard on yourself for those days or weeks when you go off track. No, you're not going to get it just right every single day; no one, not even myself, is expected to do that. That's an unrealistic objective. When we go off course we need to identify it, correct it, accept it, forgive ourselves and move on. We don't need to try to make up for overeating one day by starving the next. Just put it behind you and get back to your healthy nutrition plan the following day.

What you'll learn as you continue to read through this book is that our mindset and emotional condition directly affect our well-being. Feeling regretful and guilty is not only unnecessary, it's unhealthy. So please, go easy on yourself, apply compassion and understanding, and give yourself credit for the things you're doing right, starting here and now with the way you're focusing your time and energy to learn about healthy nutrition.

ACTION STEP

An example of a healthy day's nutrition based on my goals, preferences and schedule looks like this:

Example:

(My daily nutrition plan described on page 60.)

Someone I can share my nutrition plan with at the beginning of the week or each evening so they can help keep me accountable is:

Example:

Dietician, family member, friend from the transformation community.

Someone I can offer support, encouragement and friendly accountability to help them improve their daily nutrition is:

Example:

Friend, family member, someone from the transformation community.

CONCLUSION

The way you eat each day has the potential to significantly improve your life now and far into the future. Or, it can produce devastating consequences on your body and mind. How it goes is up to you and the choices you make. Now that you know about the 7 essential nutrients and the importance of eating the right food combinations frequently through the day, the next step is putting your knowledge into action. When you do, you'll begin to feel better immediately. By sticking with it, day after day, you'll be happy to discover that your body becomes increasingly healthy while your mind becomes brighter and more alive. Perhaps nothing is more satisfying than that.

4

The Community Connection

What's the best diet?

A group of doctors and researchers from the Department of Nutrition, Harvard School of Public Health, decided to investigate the answer to that question which is so often asked today.

They started by recruiting 800 overweight men and women between the ages of 30-70 years. They divided them into four groups. One followed a low-fat, high-protein plan; another ate low-fat, average-protein; a third group was asked to follow the high-fat, high-protein approach popularized by Dr. Atkins some years ago; and the last one ate high-fat, average-protein.

The doctors, recognizing the vital importance of coming up with effective solutions to help people reduce their weight and improve their health, worked diligently, carefully monitoring the test subjects for two years.

The final results revealed a very significant finding: All the plans worked about the same. As long as the overweight individuals in the study lowered their calorie intake, they were able to lose weight and improve their health.

The New England Journal of Medicine published the findings of this study in its prestigious journal, February 26, 2009. In reading the full report, I carefully reviewed the methods utilized in the study and looked over the data which supported the findings. It was all pretty much plain vanilla until I unexpectedly came across something that didn't make the headlines, but perhaps should have.

On the next to last page, in pretty small print, the report revealed that study participants who attended support group sessions over the course of the study lost an average of 20 lbs. Interestingly, the people who didn't attend the group meetings sustained an average weight loss of only 9 lbs at the end of the 2-year research project. That's a 225% difference! It didn't matter which eating plan they followed, if they attended the support group sessions, their results more than doubled. One of the researchers very astutely concluded that the study demonstrates effective weight management isn't a matter of finding the right macronutrient (protein, carbs, fat) combination; it's a matter of *finding the right support*. And that's what this chapter is all about.

SUPPORT GROUPS AND COMMUNITY CONNECTION

Modern science may be just beginning to discover the power of community support to help people change their lives but the tradition goes as far back as recorded history. Tribes, villages, groups of extended family, these are all examples of supportive communities which banded together to increase the group's and each individual's survival and strength.

Spiritual traditions, as far back as 3000 BC, have been found to include fellowship—worshiping with others—as a fundamental element of their practice. Fraternal organizations and governing groups have been around for ages as well. Right on up through modern religion and even science, communities of people who share beliefs and intentions tend to come together in order to embolden each person's capability as well as that of the collective group.

Right on up through a few generations ago there was still a strong sense of community in towns and cities all across America—people seldom felt alone and isolated in their experience of life. Fast-forward to right now. Large-scale studies and surveys show that nearly half the population reports that they struggle to feel like they belong to any meaningful group. Along with that statistic, people report more than a 37% drop in their perceived quality of life compared to a generation ago. In that period of time, rates of depression, overweight and obesity, anxiety, and addiction have doubled or even tripled.

Abraham Maslow, a pioneer in the science of psychology and philosopher of the human condition, wrote that 'belonging' is a fundamental human need. Without it, people feel a lack of safety and security. Contemporary neurologist, Ronald Ruden, M.D., Ph.D., has demonstrated that the human brain needs socialization and connection in order to retain a healthy chemical balance. He postulates that throughout the timeline of our ancestors' existence, they discovered survival was more likely within a group. And as such, we come from a far-reaching genetic heritage of people who lived, worked, prayed and played together.

Dr. Ruden's studies show that without sufficient community connection our brains produce less serotonin, a key neurotransmitter that gives us a feeling of security and well-being. When serotonin levels are deficient, another one of our natural chemicals, called dopamine, becomes overactive. Now dopamine is the 'gotta-have-it' neurotransmitter. It's what makes Johnny run; it's what makes us crave and strive for everything from money to sex to food and intoxicating substances. When we score one of those things, our brains release serotonin and for a short period of time we're satisfied, we're fulfilled. But then serotonin levels dip again and dopamine drives us into another cycle of craving, seeking, getting… and then over and over again.

'Bio-balance' is what the doctor calls a healthy condition of the brain. A lack of it is what produces the constant craving for something, anything, that will at least for a few moments, bring harmony and peace of mind. However, long-term bio-balance depends on one key element, perhaps more than anything else, and that is close and meaningful kinship with fellow members of the human family.

Studies show that when people are taken out of isolation and given the opportunity to form bonds and friendships with others, their bio-balance begins to restore itself in a matter of weeks. And of course, if they disconnect and isolate again, the uncontrollable cravings return.

Remember, solitary confinement is to this day, one of the harshest, legal forms of punishment that can be carried out against anyone. Unfortunately, it's one that many inflict on themselves in this modern world.

ADDICTION, RECOVERY AND SUPPORT GROUPS

With the concept of bio-balance, what we see is modern science confirming and offering explanation for something that human beings have intuited for centuries. It also helps to explain why the people in the Harvard study, who became part of a support group, had so much better results than those who didn't. The possibility of renewing bio-balance offers insight as to why one of the most important and effective treatments for addictive cravings is to connect the person who's suffering to a community of others who've shared the same or similar struggle at some point in their lives. Very often the only way to sustain recovery from alcoholism, eating disorders, and narcotic addiction, is to remain active in and connected to a community of peers.

From the findings of the research study discussed at the beginning of this chapter, it looks very much like we can include recovery from overweight and obesity on that very same list. The almost certain and astronomically high recidivism rate amongst individuals who have initial success with weight loss absolutely parallels what is seen with conditions which are more typically known as addictions.

Is being significantly overweight a physical manifestation of an inner imbalance which is resulting in classic addictive cravings? If it is, it eclipses the number of those addicted to alcohol and drugs by a landslide margin. With approximately 160 million folks in America unable to maintain a healthy weight, despite the ongoing proliferation of healthy food choices, exercise machines, and fitness centers, it sure looks to me like if people could change, they would change.

What I've discovered over the last 10 years especially is that many people who have tried and failed to sustain healthy weight loss are as trapped by their cravings as the addictive drinker is by his. This being said and realized, it becomes clear that sustaining weight loss should be looked at as a form of lifelong recovery, and as such, connecting with and participating in a support group of people dedicated to being healthy may be the single most important requirement for long-term success.

FINDING THE RIGHT SUPPORT FOR YOU

So now we know that being connected to a supportive community can help us make and even maintain important lifestyle changes in order to accomplish everything from weight loss to abstaining from life-threatening substance abuse. The question at this point is how do you determine what group is right for you. There are a couple key factors to making the right choice.

For starters, numerous studies and plenty of real-world examples show that there's something very special and powerful about being in communion with others who can relate to the adversity you might be going through. For example, studies conducted at Stanford University have shown that patients who are suffering from breast cancer, who regularly attend support groups with others facing the same condition, live significantly longer than those who do not. In the recovery community it's been proven over and over again that those with a history of substance abuse receive tremendous benefit by being in rapport with others who've experienced difficulty in life because of drugs or alcohol as well. Very much the same thing has been observed with gambling, smoking and eating disorders.

In our transformation community people have reported significantly better results when they connect and regularly communicate with people they identify with. Those who come into the transformation program with over 50 lbs of unhealthy weight they need to let go of can connect with men and women in the community who've accomplished something similar in the last year or two. Those facing diabetes, depression or compulsive cycles of negative thinking have discovered very much the same thing.

And so, very often the right support group for you is one where you can connect to many others who are going to be able to hear and understand your concerns, questions, and feelings because they've gone through it too. For example, at transformation.com, virtually everyone in the community holds a common intention which is to make healthy changes in their lives that make a difference in the lives of others. That is a powerful connector and one which allows most all of us to feel a sense of kinship and belonging. Subgroups that connect even more specifically continue to gather and gain strength as our community continues to grow.

Another key factor to keep in mind is that the true value of the community connection isn't in the short-term; it's in the long run. It's vitally important to establish yourself within a group that is easy to connect with and which you enjoy being a part of. For many, regular gatherings at the local church or community center have become a part of life for decades. For others, getting together regularly with a group of close friends for lunch or dinner is a sustainable way to stay in touch.

With the evolution of the Internet, people from around the world are forming borderless and close-knit communities with peers. This is very much what we see happening at transformation.com. The bonds become surprisingly strong and authentic, so much so that when online friends meet in person it's almost akin to a family reunion. Because people can easily access the community from any computer 24 hours a day, 7 days a week, 365 days a year, they can receive support precisely when they need it and for as long as they choose to be involved.

This is a tremendous advantage for those with busy schedules and high demands on their time and attention. In fact, studies have shown that not only do online support communities work, regular attendance and participation can go up as much as 50% compared to location-based meetings. That's not to say that in-person gatherings do not have significant value; of course, they absolutely do.

There's a powerful energy exchange which some experts believe contributes to the healing process on a cellular level between people who are going through a health challenge like cancer and those who've healthfully come out the other side. A combination of online support participation and somewhat regular in-person meeting attendance is a remarkably good way to harness the power of community connection.

Ultimately what keeps people involved in supportive communities is how much they enjoy the experience. It's hard for any of us to maintain a voluntary commitment to something we just don't find pleasant much less fun. Typically, people who are looking to make healthy, positive changes in their lives enjoy having the opportunity to connect with others who are on the same journey and share a similar positive attitude. Communities, in person or online, that devolve into cultures of complaint, cynicism and egoic immaturity don't last long, or if they do, they don't retain quality, open-hearted, intelligent and other-centered members. And as such, they become groups which enable bad behavior and unhealthy ways of thinking.

So be sure to choose a group that you enjoy being a part of and that is consistently positive, uplifting and inspiring for you.

HOW TO GIVE AND RECEIVE SUPPORT

Oftentimes making a community connection introduces us to a world that can significantly juxtapose the one we're used to living in. Healthy and helpful support groups tend to speak the language of the heart where open and honest expression of emotions supersedes telling each other what we think. For most, interactions with others in everyday life tend to involve sharing just the most basic information necessary to support interactions. In support groups, that's just not enough to benefit you or anyone else. In fact, at our transformation community there's very little interest in the superficial details of one another's lives.

Friends get to know each other at a heart-to-heart level through a process of open and ongoing sharing of our setbacks and success, our deepest hopes and fears, as well as our strengths and weaknesses. People who connect and grow to care about each other deeply in a supportive community may oftentimes not even know what kind of car you drive, what kind of salary you make, or even what credentials and titles you might use every day to identify and define you. Because of factors like these, it does take some getting used to, and that's perfectly normal.

When first introduced to a new and supportive community, many find it helpful to sit back and observe for a day or two while they learn the patterns of interaction within the group culture. From there, getting involved is the next step and one that I just absolutely encourage everyone to take.

Start by introducing yourself and sharing your intentions and goals. When you do this at transformation.com, I guarantee you will be very pleasantly surprised by the warm welcome you are given and the numerous, sincere offers of assistance. If you ever find yourself in a community that doesn't respond this way to your introduction, please reconsider if that's the right group for you.

As your comfort and trust levels increase, you'll want to become more in-volved in the giving and receiving of support. Every member of the group has something valuable to offer and every contribution is appreciated by others within the community. Primarily what we each have to share that means the most is our life experience.

Why have you decided to be a part of the support group? Most always it's because you want to change something about yourself—to better yourself. That's something to be proud of and is a wonderfully authentic thing to share again and again. Every time you do you'll be communicating something very tangible and meaningful that others can connect to.

Again, this is in pretty significant opposition to what we're accustomed to in the fast-paced everyday world of our modern environment. I've known some people for over twenty years and I still don't know what their aspira-tions are or what they really care about. And without something more to go on—something authentic and from the heart—there just isn't very much of a significant connection. On the other hand, when we get to know each other at a deeper level, which it's surprisingly easy to do, even online, the friendships are remarkably rich.

In fact, the more you share, the more others can support you. And the more open you are, the more you'll receive the same in return. Make no mis-take, it's a very special and incredibly meaningful experience to be allowed into another person's life. Just being a completely nonjudgmental, uncondi-tionally caring witness to another's revelations and personal discoveries is incredibly healing, for both the sender and receiver.

When people share their goals and challenges with one another, they can immediately determine, at a very intuitive level, how they can support each other's positive growth and evolution and help keep each other accountable in a friendly, compassionate way. What I've discovered over the years is that the best accountability partner you can have is someone who is actively and earnestly in pursuit of his or her personal goals, just like you are doing the work to achieve yours. You see, this builds mutual respect, and that's just not something which happens when efforts to hold someone accountable become authoritative, sometimes disingenuous, and delivered by someone who's not walking the walk.

When accountability is mutual, it's most often well received and can literally become a make-or-break aspect of sticking with any challenging program of life change, transformation included. I highly recommend that if you don't have an accountability partner yet, that you openly and specifically share your intentions and goals with others and make a connection with someone who's open and willing to do the same.

THE HEART CONNECTION

Fascinating new scientific discoveries in the field of subtle energies show that the heart does indeed have its own language, which is expressed in electromagnetic waves. In fact, one research project at the HeartMath Institute in northern California revealed that the energy of the heart is 5,000 times that of the brain. And so when two or more people connect and communicate with a relaxed and open mind (as opposed to a rigid, opinionated and judgmental one), their hearts begin to synchronize. When this happens, both people can become more aligned with a healthy vibrational frequency or energy. This is especially true if at least one of the people in the group is in a good, healthy, loving place.

Again, it seems that spiritual traditions had it right long ago when they would 'prescribe' participation in what's called a 'speaking circle' to cure conditions ranging from common influenza to fear and anxiety. Native American Indians, in particular, were known for their healing ceremonies. When anyone in the tribe was ailing, they were invited to sit within a circle of fellows and simply talk about what they were experiencing.

Those sitting in the circle would listen with all of their intention focused on the moment. They would calm their minds and listen and receive with their hearts open, acknowledging what was said. They wouldn't try to fix the person, as they believed that their own thinking would be an insufficient cure; they merely sat in the circle, with inner stillness. They had complete faith that the group's meditation and prayer would facilitate a flow of life from the Great Spirit, through their hearts and into the ailing member of their tribe. They would remain in the circle until the person became well.

Today this ritual is still alive and well and is practiced in supportive communities around the world. A large or small number (two or more) of group members arrange chairs in a circle, with no one and nothing in the center, they then proceed to go around the circle with each person sharing what's in their heart for around 2-4 minutes. Each person is asked to share their authentic feelings. Those forming the circle remain nonjudgmental, open, caring and fully present. Oftentimes people come into the circle frazzled and stressed. For many, that state is one that often triggers unhealthy habits like overeating or drinking. After sitting in the circle for a time, their energy is often transformed into a state of loving peacefulness.

Speaking circles can also be very effectively utilized for making a shift into a deep state of gratitude. In this instance, each member of the circle would speak for a few minutes about what they're thankful for; going beyond the superficial and again, into their heart of hearts while communicating. By the end of the ritual virtually everyone who has participated undergoes a kind of spiritual and energetic shift into a state of harmony, health, even bliss.

As a regular participant and facilitator of these kinds of groups I can attest to the profound effects they've had on my own health and happiness. I can also highly recommend that if you have the opportunity to participate, jump at it. Speaking circles are often held at local transformation gatherings. You can find a directory of local groups on transformation.com.

ACTION STEP:

Three people I can count on for unconditional, nonjudgmental support throughout my transformation are:

Example: *Best friend, spouse, transformation community member.*

Someone I can call at 3:00 AM to share something which is weighing on my heart is:

Example: *Family member, counselor, very special friend from your personal life or the transformation community.*

Someone who is working to achieve their transformation goals whom I can count on to keep me accountable, in a caring and respectful way, and encourage me to do the work I need to do to achieve the results I'm working towards is:

Example: *Friend or fellow member of the transformation community.*

A support group that I can be an active participant in to give and receive heart-centered support and encouragement is:

Example: *Local church group, recovery group, or a support group on transformation.com.*

A community where I feel a sense of belonging and kinship with others because of our common intentions is:

Example: *Your town, your neighborhood (if you have a strong sense of community there), church, where you work, or transformation.com.*

Three people who can count on me for unconditional and nonjudgmental support, anytime and no matter what are:

Example: *A parent, brother, sister, child, co-worker, friend, someone from the transformation community.*

CONCLUSION

Do ancient rituals like the ones discussed in this text actually facilitate divine healing? Or do they restore bio-balance in the brain through socialization and closeness with others as the neurologists contend? Or does healing take place by actually strengthening the electromagnetic energy flow to and from the heart?

It's hard to say for sure. Future scientific studies and discoveries may eventually lead to a conclusive answer; for now, what we do know for sure is that open and caring communication within a supportive community has the very real potential to empower everyone to make and sustain healthy and meaningful changes in their lives.

No matter how you look at it—from a scientific, spiritual or psychological point of view—making the community connection can be a powerful source of healing and positive change.

5

Lifetime Intentions

What is the ultimate purpose of your life? What is it that you feel, in your heart, that you're meant to accomplish while you're here?

Very often, when I ask people these two questions, they go silent. Then their eyes look up, down, back up and around while their head tilts and they say, *"Well... um... hmm... my purpose?"* It's like they're looking for something in their thoughts which they know is there, but just can't seem to locate.

On the other hand, we can rattle off trivial details from the popular culture at the drop of a hat. For example, who's the favorite on American Idol this week, which team won the ballgame last night, who's the most talked about celebrity this week. Others can tell you all about the latest fluctuations and trends in the stock market, what the hot debate going on in Congress right now is and what the next big breakthrough in technology is going to be. Virtually everyone in the mainstream has a pulse on some aspect of what's happening in the external world.

Unfortunately, when it comes to ourselves—our interior world—the vast majority know very little. "What is my life all about? Why do I do what I do? What direction is my life going?" Who's got time to answer questions like that when there are over 200 television shows on every minute of the day, millions of websites to review, and you've got Yahoo on your Blackberry. The deeper questions of life have been put on the back burner so we can have time for the seemingly more urgent things like Tweeting, texting, Skyping, Googling, and poking our friends on Facebook.

It all becomes so consuming that we end up merely skimming the surface of what our lives are truly all about. And as a result, life becomes more and more superficial and mundane. It's very likely that it will remain that way until we make the time and put in the effort to discover something richer, more purposeful, more real.

Again, I ask: *What is the ultimate purpose of your life? What is it that you feel, in your heart, that you're meant to accomplish in the time you're here?*

Ideally, we should not only be able to quickly answer those two questions with crystal clarity, but the way we live our everyday lives should speak to them also. You see, the ultimate purpose of your life is more about how you live it than anything else. What kind of work you do, what titles you earn, what roles you play, are of secondary importance.

When you do the work to clearly identify and understand what your life's mission is all about and what your aim is, it can act as a beacon—a light that guides your everyday decisions such as what to do with your time, energy, and abilities. That focal point can become a source of resilience. No matter what the setback or adversity, having an absolute certainty about your purpose will pick you back up and motivate you to continue on in the right direction.

When you don't truly know what your life's mission is, you're in danger of taking off in the wrong direction. This is a mistake many people make when they jump in and start making changes in their lives, selecting goals or destinations, without having a meaningful, long-range vision for where they're going. After months, even years, of continuing on in that direction, they might reach the top, take a deep breath, open their eyes, look across the horizon and realize, "Son of a biscuit… I climbed the wrong mountain!"

How do we avoid this common mistake? Well, there's a very good way to take a look at whether or not you're on the right path. It begins with a little detective work and soul searching. What you'll be looking for is your 'True North.' It's the direction your life was intended to go, from the beginning. How do you find it? That's what this chapter is all about.

FOLLOW YOUR HEART

Questions of purpose are answered in the language of the heart: inspiration, joyfulness, enthusiasm, gratitude. So now I ask: When have you felt the most inspired, happy, energized and complete during your life? What kind of work were you doing, and more importantly, *how* were you doing it? Were you pouring your heart and soul into it? What kind of pursuits and endeavors engage you at that level, so much so that you feel like you could do them for long hours, only to be more energetic (not drained) as a result?

Maybe you think the world would be a better place if more people generously shared their blessings with those less fortunate? If so, how can you embody those qualities—how can you be that change you want to see in the world? If you believe all people—white or black, rich or poor, male or female—should be treated equally, then treat everyone with equality and fairness. Would you like to see the world filled with more compassion and kindness? If so, become happier and more caring.

That's how simple this all can be. For me, when I'm aligned with my purposeful vision I feel lighter, more alive and I lose track of time. It's the kind of thing that I don't even care if I get paid for. Writing this chapter, here and now, is on that list for me because helping people transform their lives is something that I have relentless enthusiasm for—it's an aspect of my purpose. What comes to mind for you? Do you light up when you're around kids or animals or out in nature? Does the life energy and inspiration flow when you're creating something?

When you're doing what you're made to do, you'll know it. There's a unique state of mind and emotion that you'll be in; it's a feeling like no other. When we're in that 'zone' it's a remarkable time of healing where the immune system is strengthened, stress dissipates; worry and fear are replaced with confidence and love.

> **"Don't worry what the world needs, ask what makes you**
> **come alive and do that. Because what the world needs are**
> **people who have come alive."** - *Howard Thurman*

It might not be so much about finding the 'perfect career'—remember it's how we do what we do that expresses purpose. A waitress who finds meaning in helping bring love and happiness to others can absolutely let that intention flow by how she does her job. If helping other people get healthy is meaningful to you, you can fulfill that by being the healthiest person you can be inside and out. And you can do that regardless of whether you're working as an architect, manager, merchant or Marine.

Consider these questions and talk about them with your spouse, friends or fellow members of the transformation community, and at the end of the chapter I'll ask you to write your answers down. By doing this you're going to become more aware of how you can live your purpose in everyday life.

BEGIN AT THE END

Okay, now try this: Let's say you and I are having a conversation many years from now. We're old and gray but healthy and wise. We're sitting on the patio of your beautiful home, watching the summer sunset. You've got a sparkle in your eye and this wonderfully warm, authentic smile which rises up from within. It's clear that somewhere along the way you identified and answered your heart's calling. You aligned your thoughts, actions and objectives with that purpose, and as such, your life has become free from worry, regret and resentment. You're looking back at the time between then and now.

I'm excited to hear your story and I ask, "Why are you so grateful, happy, healthy, and content?" You smile and begin to tell me all about it. What do you say? Consider it and in just a bit I'm going to ask you to write that script.

COMPARE AND CONTRAST

Alright, now I want you to look forward out into the future and consider an altogether different scenario. This time, I've come to see you because I received news that you don't have much more time to live. My heart is breaking while you tell me how you wish you would have changed when you had the opportunity. You explain that you never thought life would go by so fast or that this would happen to you. The Monday you said you were going to start to turn it all around... well, it never came. What makes this even harder to hear is that I knew all along you had every bit as much potential to be healthy, happy, and fulfill your purpose as anyone else.

Imagine that you are there now looking back. What are your most painful regrets? What were your biggest mistakes? What do you wish you would have done differently? Think about it... and in a few moments I'm going to ask you to write that script also.

CLARIFYING YOUR LIFETIME INTENTIONS

By answering the questions above, you're going to gain a whole new awareness about what's important to you, what gives you inspiration and energy, and also what you feel you really need to accomplish in the time you're here. And not only that, you're going to make these discoveries in time to do something about them. This is all very good and exciting news!

The next step in this process is to carefully compose your personal mission statement which outlines your lifetime intentions. In this decree you'll clarify and document what it's all about for you. It will reveal the ultimate purpose of your life, as you know it now. It will express what you feel in your heart you're meant to accomplish while you're here. This statement will become a beacon of light which gives you direction and lets you know which goals are most worthy of pursuing and which mountains you need to climb. It can guide your daily decisions, and according to many wise teachers, stating your lifetime intentions with confidence and clarity can invoke powers beyond the individual self to help you manifest the life you're envisioning.

> **"The moment one definitely commits oneself, then Providence moves too. All sorts of things occur to help one that would never otherwise have occurred."** - *Goethe*

Much has been written and said about the somewhat mystical power that earnest intentions seem to hold. Throughout the wisdom of the ages and in spiritual traditions all over the world, people were taught that intention (essentially a form of prayer), particularly when it's focused on something that serves the greater good (not just our own self-interests), serendipitously alters the future. Good intentions that one is committed to and takes action towards seem to have a way of opening doors which were previously closed. These intentions can attract the right people and resources to help you fulfill them. They also somehow seem to summon renewed energy and strength.

Intentions are not just thoughts. They're the powerful, purposeful reasons which come from deep within our heart and soul. When we hear about universal principles such as 'the law of attraction,' it's important to know that it's the force of intention, not merely thought, that can metaphorically move mountains. Thoughts come and go; in fact, most people's thoughts change every six seconds according to scientific studies. Intention is different; it's there all the time. And the more clear, focused and specific it is, the greater its effects will be.

On the surface, this hardly seems to make sense and is often scoffed at by those who see it merely as 'wishful thinking.' I'd probably see it the same way if I hadn't opened my mind and done the necessary and legitimate research required to gain an understanding of it. Scientific studies, going back a few decades, do in fact exist which demonstrate that prayer and intention have power. They can alter circumstances and promote healing. More recently, Dr. Gary Schwartz, at the University of Arizona, and Lynne McTaggart, author of *The Field* and *The Intention Experiment*, have demonstrated through scientifically valid studies that what people want or intend to have happen can have far-reaching effects on the physical world. Those effects are even more powerful when a group of people hold the same or similar intention.

Dr. Schwartz's studies have demonstrated that people on one side of the country intending something to happen in a lab, thousands of miles away, on the other side of the country, cause the behavior of matter to change. These kinds of effects are called 'nonlocal phenomenon' and explaining how they work is the stuff of quantum physics. Brilliant researchers including Max Planck, Albert Einstein, Niels Bohr, Roger Penrose, Stuart Hameroff and others have dedicated a significant part of their life's work to understanding, explaining, and developing practical applications for this field of science.

Intention has significant effects at the local level too, right here in our physical bodies. Researchers at the Institute of Cognitive Neuroscience recently reported their investigations show that when people hold positive, life-affirming intentions, their brains become healthier. Clarifying your personal mission and purpose, committing to it, and taking action in that direction may therefore help you build a better, healthier brain, which in turn will directly support your efforts to improve your life.

Fortunately, you don't have to completely understand how all that works in order to benefit from it. You simply need to do the work to become clear about what's most important to you and then state your intentions.

ACTION STEP:

I feel inspired, energetic, confident, and alive when I'm engaged in these three activities:

Example:

1) Helping people become healthier and happier.

2) Taking care of my own health by exercising and eating right.

3) Working hard and being productive in service to others.

Moving my awareness into the future, seeing myself when I'm old and gray, healthy and wise, the answer I'll give to explain why I'm so grateful, happy, healthy, and content is:

Example:

The reason I'm feeling so good is because many years ago I made the decision to live my life in a healthy way. I found that when I take good care of myself I have more strength and energy to share with others. Ever since, I've held the intention of making healthy changes in my life that make a difference in the lives of others, and that path has led me to this point.

Looking at the other side, envisioning my future life as unhealthy and unfulfilling, my most painful regrets would be:

Example:

My single-most painful regret would be that I didn't live a healthy life. I wasted too much time procrastinating and making excuses. I mistakenly assumed that I would be healthy far into the future, even though I wasn't doing anything to ensure it. I wish I would have learned more, loved more, cared more. I would regret not having done something meaningful to make a difference in the lives of others.

This is my mission statement which clarifies my lifetime intentions:

Example:

My lifetime intentions are to help people, to fulfill my potential, to live an active and healthy life, to embrace change, accept challenges, confront fear, experience the world, know myself, grow spiritually, live with a clear mind, an open heart and to gratefully enjoy it all.

THIS IS AN ONGOING PROCESS

Keep in mind that your statement of lifetime intentions is going to be a 'living document.' By that I mean it will evolve and grow as you do throughout your transformation journey. Be sure to read what you've written and contemplate it, perhaps every week. Also, ask yourself often if you are living in alignment with your stated intentions. If not, what do you need to change? As time goes by and your life unfolds, feel free to modify your personal mission statement as appropriate.

CONCLUSION

We're all here for a reason. Each of us has unique abilities, strengths, and talents that we were given to help us accomplish our purpose in life. Unfortunately, most people don't give the matter much thought. There are so many other things that distract our attention in this microchip-driven modern world. However, when you make the time to find the answers within, your life will take on new meaning. It becomes easier to make decisions because your purpose points you in the right direction. The more you align with your lifetime intentions, the happier, healthier, and more fulfilling your life will be.

6

Healthy Spaces Makeover

"What we surround ourselves with we tend to become."

A quick story: Last summer I was giving a presentation to a group of businessmen at a seminar in Los Angeles. The topic was how to live a healthy, long, successful life. I asked them a series of short questions in an effort to learn a little more about them. First, "How many of you have been to a bar?" Everybody in the room raised their hand. "How many of you have had a beer in a bar?" Almost all hands went up. Then I asked, "How many of you have been to a church?" The majority confirmed that they had. "How many of you have had a beer in a church?" No hands were raised, and from the stage I could feel their collective chuckle.

This simple and lighthearted demonstration always illustrates an important insight. And that is, the very same person will do two completely different things depending on the environment they're in. That's what I want to talk to you about today: your environment. How it can support healthy behavior or do the opposite.

87

What we're going to do now is take a good, honest look at the overall environment you are in each day. From there, we'll determine which aspects of it are working for you and which might be working against you. Then I'll guide you through some action steps that will help you make some positive changes starting right away.

When I say *environment* I'm referring to the *people* we interact with, the *places* we go and the spaces we live and work in, as well as the *things* around us at home and work especially.

PEOPLE

The people in our environment have a powerful effect on our energy, thoughts, emotions and health. In fact, what I've noticed over the years is that healthy, happy people tend to have healthy, happy friends. And it's no coincidence either. The people we choose to share our time with are always influenced by the direction of our lives, and we can't help but be influenced by the direction of theirs. It's important to recognize this fact. And get this: Not only are we connected to our friends and family members when we're face to face, but according to breakthrough scientific findings in the field of quantum physics and nonlocality, we even share thoughts and emotions with them when we're far apart.

It's true. Researchers have performed extensive studies which show that the minds of people who communicate regularly become 'entangled' (that's the scientific term) and in sync, no matter how close or far apart they are from one another. This phenomenon may very well be the source of certain synchronicities that most all of us are familiar with. For example, where the phone rings and you know exactly who's calling before you even say "Hello." Where you can feel that a family member or friend, from across the country, is having an incredibly exciting day or perhaps not doing well, even before you're notified by phone or email.

Let's consider that for a moment: If the energy of our thoughts and intentions affect those we're close to, and if what's on their minds and in their hearts has an influence on us, what does that mean? For starters, it seems to highlight the importance of doing all we can to be healthy and inspired in order to have a positive impact on the lives of our friends and family members. Also, if someone around you is suffering from an illness, it appears that one of the ways you can help them heal is to take good care of yourself.

You see, your well-being is shared with everyone you come into contact with. Maybe you've even experienced this firsthand where just being around a certain person has made you feel brighter and happier. This happens all the time within the support groups at transformation.com and it seems to help explain why so many people start feeling better and more energetic the day they become actively involved.

Now let's take a look at what to do when some of the folks we're around are not in a healthy, positive place. We can all find ourselves off track from time to time, but when people are chronically complaining, criticizing others, not taking care of themselves, and they've been that way for quite a while, with no real intention of making a change, it's a reason for concern. These are the type of people who, when you talk to them for any length of time, leave you feeling drained and wiped out. It's not that they're inherently bad people, they're just in a bad place, and until they become open and willing to change, their condition will continue to persist.

It's an unfortunate truth that in order for you to make the healthy transformation you've decided to make, you might need to limit contact with them when possible, and instead spend more time in rapport with people who are on a good path. As we discussed in a previous chapter, being part of a supportive community, where people are focused on improving their lives, is a healthy environment for certain. Even communicating for just a few minutes a day with a positive person or two can be a big help.

Of course, I realize that in some cases with family members or co-workers we might not have much of an option as to how often we're around them. In these cases, it's important that we learn to accept that each person is at their own place on the path, and it does little to no good to resist that or try to change them. If and when they reach the point where they're ready and willing, they will very often ask you for help, especially if you're the living example of how transformation can improve your body and life.

PLACES

Where we live, where we work and the places we go are also part of our environment. Each one influences our behavior and health for the better or worse, and they can even affect our thought processes, energy and mood. For example, have you ever walked into a room where people were arguing and then walked out in a different mental and emotional condition than before? Experiences like that are not uncommon. What's even more interesting is that some people can walk into that same room, after the angry people have left, and still be affected by the energy.

Likewise, have you ever walked into a place and noticed your mind felt brighter and calmer and your heart seemed to be more open and loving? I know I sure have. While traveling around the world this past decade, I visited many sacred sites in Europe, the Mediterranean and the Far East. Perhaps the most inspiring man-made place of all was the Sistine Chapel in Vatican City. The moment you step into the chapel you become filled with what I can only describe as a warm and loving spiritual energy that very nearly takes your breath away.

Gazing at Michelangelo's brilliant fresco on the ceiling and his paintings on the walls, which depict the story of Genesis and The Last Judgment, is a life-changing experience I'll never forget. I could imagine that the energy of that place could heal body, mind and soul.

And the creepiest place I ever spent the night was in a hotel in Germany. After being there for 10 hours, I felt like the life force had just been drained from my body. A couple weeks after I stayed there, I learned that the hotel was constructed over an old POW camp.

My favorite spot in the natural world, out of all the places I've been, is a tie between the Greek island Santorini (Plato's Atlantis) and my favorite perch on a hill overlooking the beautiful blue Pacific Ocean on the southwest corner of Maui. I'm convinced both locations have healing power.

Now those are dramatic examples, I realize, but they've taught me, by direct experience, the power different places have on us. In more subtle ways we experience this every day. And becoming aware of that allows us to make conscious decisions about where we spend our time.

THINGS

There's no place like home for getting healthy. That is, if it's organized and filled with things that nourish your well-being. But far too often, the place where we live is part of the problem. When it's a cluttered mess, with a kitchen filled with sugary, processed, high-calorie foods, it interferes with both mental clarity and physical health.

That's why one of the first things I do when I begin working with someone new is meet them at their home to do what I call a 'Healthy Spaces Makeover.' I start in the kitchen by opening the cabinets and refrigerator and I take a photo of each. Then I get out a Hefty trash bag and I go to work. Out goes the half-eaten box of sugary cereal, the leftover potato chips, cookies, Pop Tarts, sodas, ice cream and such. Everything that's packed with empty calories and practically devoid of essential nutrients must go. Then it's off to the grocery store to stock up on fresh fruits and vegetables, brown rice, oatmeal, lean sources of protein like salmon, chicken, eggs, protein powder, light yogurt and low-fat cottage cheese, as well as plenty of pure water.

Then it's back to the kitchen where we put these new items in the cabinets and refrigerator. Then I take another photo and I paste it, as well as the photo taken before, on a sheet of paper. The before and after comparison is often very dramatic—like the difference between night and day. In just a matter of a few short hours, we change the kitchen from a health hazard to a vibrant source of great energy. I tape the sheet of paper with both photos on a cabinet near the refrigerator so the person has a crystal-clear example of how I need that kitchen to look from this point forward, throughout the 18-week transformation process.

MORE THINGS

Beyond the kitchen, most of us have more things around the house than we know what to do with. When our bedroom, home office, and living space become a cluttered mess, it can weigh us down and even interfere with focused thinking. The accumulation of more and more things, especially the ones that are not useful or valued, can form a kind of 'psychic debris' which often makes us feel on the inside the way it looks on the outside. And it seems to have this effect even when you're not around it.

The solution, again, is a Healthy Spaces Makeover where we take action to clear the clutter, getting rid of things we don't need in order to create a more focused and pleasant space. After the kitchen, I'll often come back in a week to help renew another room. I've helped turn many cluttered basements, spare bedrooms and garages into really nice home gyms. I'm sure you've done this kind of 'spring cleaning' at various times in the past, and maybe you can even attest to how much better it makes you feel. What we want is for the environment you live in to be the healthiest, most nurturing of all. But if you're not there now, it requires some focused, conscious mental and physical effort to get there.

MUSIC AND TV PROGRAMMING ARE THINGS

Did you know that experts in measuring the body's reaction to music can determine whether the sounds are strengthening or weakening you? To make their determination, they use the same kind of evaluations that doctors utilize to find out what people are allergic to. What they're discovering is that some forms of music, such as Beethoven's Symphonies, increase almost everyone's mental performance on various quizzes and tests, as well as their balance, hand-eye coordination and muscle strength. They've also discovered that certain kinds of aggressive music have the opposite effect.

TV programming can also produce a significant effect on our state of being. Scenes that feature violence and negativity increase blood pressure, activate adrenalin which causes our heart rate to go up, while also stimulating the fear centers of the brain. This in turn can release a hormone called cortisol. When cortisol is produced in excess amounts, it can cause damage to blood and brain cells as well as contribute to the buildup of weight gain, especially around the midsection.

Not only that, but whenever we experience stress we're more likely to reach for something to make us feel better; oftentimes that's high-sugar or high-fat comfort foods. For many others, when stress levels become uncomfortable, they reach for a cigarette or drink.

On the other hand, TV programming and videos that include inspirational content, such as examples of courage and compassion, can lower your blood pressure and heart rate while calming the mind. A Harvard University study revealed that positive programming has another health-enhancing benefit. A scientific study of a group of students who watched a video of Mother Teresa helping the needy in Calcutta revealed that immediately after viewing, the strength of their immune systems was significantly improved, compared to a group of students who didn't watch the video. These kinds of discoveries bring to light something that many of us have intuited or experienced, which is that abrasive programs can negatively impact our emotions and mindset. And over time, this can adversely affect our overall health.

It's with this awareness that I continue to executive produce inspiring, life-affirming videos, which you can find on transformation.com. Watching one of these short films first thing in the morning or right before you go to sleep at night can help put you in a positive, empowered state of mind. Please don't underestimate how much of an effect what you watch can have on you.

ACTION STEP:

Three places which empower and support my efforts to become healthier and happier are:

Example:

1) Spiritual center/church.

2) A garden, park, or other natural setting outdoors where I can enjoy fresh air and sunshine.

3) The fresh fruit section of a grocery store (rather than the drive thru at a fast-food joint).

A place I've recently been that does not support my transformation intentions and which I need to steer clear of in the future is:

Example:

A nightclub, bar or all-you-can-eat buffet.

Three people I can stay in contact with throughout this transformation program who will have a positive influence on me are:

Example:

1) Friend who's also committed to making healthy changes.

2) Doctor or counselor.

3) Supportive and optimistic spouse.

A person, or the kind of people, who may not empower or support my efforts to transform is:

Example:

Drinking buddy or anyone who's quite negative and not changing.

A place I can do a Healthy Spaces Makeover this week is:

Example:

Kitchen cabinets and refrigerator.

CONCLUSION

The people, places and things that make up our environment always have a profound effect, for better or worse, on our state of health. When you make the resolute decision to change your life for the better, it's vitally important that you take steps to cultivate the very best, healthiest environment that you possibly can. When you do, you'll find that staying on the right path throughout this journey becomes second nature.

7

Progress Not Perfection

O ver the years, I've seen far too many people give up on themselves because they simply couldn't see how well they were actually doing. An example is a gal who had become 15 pounds lighter over a period of just 8 weeks, and she was feeling better too. But in her mind, she wasn't getting anywhere at all. I asked exactly what her goal was. She explained it was to develop a perfect body, like a swimsuit model on the cover of a magazine. And she associated all of these perfect feelings she would have, once she got there.

This became her exclusive focus and each day she'd get up, look in the mirror and notice, "I'm not there yet." She didn't even see that she was making terrific progress. All she noticed was that she still didn't meet this ideal of perfection. She convinced herself she had failed, and from there, she quit. What happened was she got caught in 'The Void.'

The Void is a dangerous place we can wander into if we measure our progress based on what hasn't happened rather than what has. The Void can zap

97

your self-confidence and send your self-esteem tumbling, making it impossible for you to feel good about yourself. Hanging out there can also lead to full-time frustration, which can permeate every aspect of your life.

This painful place is a psychological purgatory where we constantly compare ourselves to an unattainable and vague ideal. This is also called 'perfectionism.' The amount of stress and suffering this causes in America today is significantly underestimated.

In a culture like ours, where the mass media continually presents pictures of so-called perfection in marketing, movies and magazines, it's difficult to feel like we're ever good enough. In a race to keep up with the Joneses, there's constant comparison and almost always a focus on what's missing, what we're not, what we need, what we're supposed to be, do, say and become. And of course, in reality, the perfect persons' lives and families really don't even exist.

The ideal is an illusion, and pursuing it is like chasing the pot of gold at the end of a rainbow—whenever you go to where it appears to be, it's always someplace else. If we continue to pursue this mirage, we are setting ourselves up for a lifetime of never feeling complete; never feeling good enough, smart enough, healthy enough, successful or beautiful enough.

Fortunately, there's a solution. There's a mindset that allows you to steer clear of The Void, while enjoying ever-increasing levels of authentic self-confidence, self-worth and fulfillment. The key is creating a game we can win.

How do we win so we can feel confident and empowered every day? Well, that happens when we make this dramatic shift where we surrender the pursuit of perfection and instead focus on progress. To do that we must stop measuring ourselves by what we haven't accomplished and start paying attention to what we have.

Whereas the ideal is always abstract and impossible to specifically define, pursuing progress becomes something altogether different, because it's clear, tangible, and objectively verifiable. Progress is a step in the right direction; it's any action you can take which moves you further away from your point A (where you were at the beginning of this process) and closer to your point B (where you decided you wanted to go).

Of course, you clarified back at the end of Chapter 1 precisely where you're beginning, as well as where you're going. I want to emphasize again that the objectives you're working towards must be stated specifically, using parameters that are objectively verifiable. For example, "Within 18 weeks, I will become 35 lbs lighter." That's clear, measurable, objectively verifiable. On the other hand, "I want to get in great shape" is not a goal; it's an ideal. It's vague and subjective. It's an example of a pseudo-goal which can lead you into The Void. We must steer clear of those kinds of targets. So please, make sure your goals in that first action step are not ideals. Please revise your goals now if necessary.

When you begin to focus on making progress, one day at a time, towards your goals, you'll discover that you don't have to wait 12 or 18 weeks to really start feeling good about yourself. You can do it every day, starting now. When you do, you'll find that the self-critiquing will fade away. Instead, you will truly see and appreciate your progress all along the way; that's something that will give you a positive focus and sense of achievement.

Focusing on your progress is not complicated at all. You simply identify actions you can take each day that will help you move towards your goals. For example, if your goal is to become 35 lbs lighter over a period of 18 weeks, you can take a step in that direction by doing 40 minutes of vigorous exercise between now and this time tomorrow. You can also avoid junk food while eating nutritious meals that provide your body with the nutrients it needs without the calories it doesn't. Another step in the right direction, which you can accomplish by the end of the day tomorrow, is offering support and encouragement to someone who is making good, healthy changes in their life too.

When you shift your focus in this way, what you'll notice, and this is a very important point, is that you will begin measuring your progress in *actions*, not results. Remember, you've got 18 weeks to accomplish the goals you decided to achieve. Like ascending from the base to the summit, the way you get there is one step at a time. If we don't recognize each step forward as progress, we begin to notice the impatient child in us asking, "Are we there yet? *Are we there yet?!*" We do a workout and then get on the scale, expecting to see results. We might stand in front of the mirror and notice we don't look like that model on the magazine cover yet. This is a game you shouldn't even play because it's one you can't win.

Without putting what you learn here into action, don't be surprised if your mind plays a trick on you where, more often than not, it will seem like you're getting nowhere. From my extensive experience in helping people through this process, I've learned that this is the number one reason why people give up, give in and quit. And sometimes they do it on the two-yard line. It's like they've gone all this way and come so close to the goal, but they can't see it and throw in the towel. I don't want that to happen to you. So please, focus on progress, not perfection.

ACTION STEP:

Five things I can do between now and the end of the day tomorrow that move me in the direction of my goals and intentions are:

Example:

1) Exercise intensely for 40 minutes.

2) Eat six nutritious meals that are nutrient rich and calorie sparse.

3) Encourage someone else who's also making healthy changes.

4) Check in with my community support group.

5) Restock my kitchen with a dozen healthy fruits and vegetables.

 100

I often call the list that you just made a 'Win List.' And what I do at the end of each day is look it over and write 'Win!' next to each action item that I followed through with. I've been doing this for years, and even to this day I smile and feel good every time I write down 'Win!' After I acknowledge and enjoy my progress for the day, I write out the next day's action items. Remember, we want to develop the good habit of paying attention to the things we're doing each day that are helping us become healthier and more energetic.

CONCLUSION

Now is the time to begin focusing on progress rather than perfection. When you do, your mindset will quickly change, and you'll gain confidence and momentum with each new day. And because this is a game you can win, you'll enjoy one victory after another. You will free yourself from living in The Void, that state of mind which leaves so many feeling incomplete and disempowered. When you approach your transformation journey this way, you may very well discover that your daily progress becomes its own reward.

8

The Big Forgive

"I met him five years after the tragedy. And it took many hours of consideration, because you don't know how you're going to react when you come face to face with your son's... with your child's killer," explains Azim Khamisa.

"I remember looking into his eyes for a very long time, trying to find a murderer in him that I could be angry with. But I didn't see a murderer in him. I looked in his eyes and I saw another soul, much like me, much like you." Azim asked for and was granted permission to visit the imprisoned, former teenage gang member who murdered his 20-year-old son Tariq, then a student at San Diego State University.

"What I saw in this tragedy was that my son was the victim of the gang member and that the gang member was a victim of society. We've created this society. So I felt as an American I must take my share of the responsibility for the bullet that took my son's life. I am Azim Khamisa, and I forgave my son's killer."

103

This remarkable father's courageous act of compassion displays an ability that most might find hard to fathom. He's given the matter much thought.

"You know you think about it… why have some important real estate of your psyche occupied with somebody who has hurt you? Why not forgive and release that real estate so love and joy can live there."

Azim continues, "Not all of us have to reach out to the family of our son's killer, or to our child's killer. Very often the issues are divorce, anger with business partners, family disagreements, all kinds of situations in our society that you can reach out and forgive, but do it with love and compassion. It's important to acknowledge our feelings and there's a lot of emotions to work through. We need to reach the point where we give up all the resentment and let it go. There's a saying, 'Resentment is like drinking poison and waiting for your enemy to die,' and I believe that."

Profound insight from a man who seemingly has every reason to see things in just the opposite light. His forgiveness isn't just lip service. It's from the heart.

"We regularly communicate by letter. He didn't really have a father. He was born to a 15 year old. I have kind of taken the father role to him." Khamisa reaches over to unfold a letter from the man he's forgiven and begins to read, "I'm writing you to wish you a happy Father's Day." He's deeply moved by the sentiment.

This forgiving father has since quit his job as a successful international investment banker to work full time in the foundation named after his son, the Tariq Khamisa Foundation. Its mission is to break the cycle of youth violence by teaching the principles of non-violence, forgiveness and peacemaking. So far, the foundation has reached over eight million at-risk youths with its inspiring message.

His son's killer is up for parole in 2027. When asked if he'll be there for him when he gets out he responds, "Absolutely. I actually offered him a job when I met him. I forgave him but I also told him, 'When you come out, you have a job at the foundation.' And we look forward to that day when he can join us because I know that he would save many more lives."

WHAT IS FORGIVENESS?

Forgiveness is a process of letting go of a resentment or grudge held against another person. "I forgive you" means "I release you." By releasing someone, we in turn are liberated from the mental, emotional and spiritual injury caused by our own pent-up, negative energy.

The word 'forgive' implies, by its components, a kind of 'giving.' And that's a very important point. You see, granting someone true forgiveness is not based on any conditions. The forgiven don't have to deserve it or earn it. It's an act of grace and mercy on your part.

Most of the world's religions include teachings on forgiveness, especially the Abrahamic faiths (Christianity, Judaism, Islam). For example, in the sacred narratives of the New Testament, Jesus (taken literally or metaphorically) said, "And when you stand praying, if you hold anything against anyone, forgive him, so that your Father in heaven may forgive your sins. But if you do not forgive, neither will your Father who is in heaven forgive your sins." (Mark 11:25-26 [NIV])

Philosophers throughout the ages have taken note of the importance of forgiveness, and some of history's most thoughtful writers have recorded their insights as well. "To err is human; to forgive is divine," wrote the eighteenth century English poet Alexander Pope.

In more recent times, particularly the last few years, the scientific community has recognized the 'medicinal value' of forgiveness. For example, in one study at Stanford University it was shown that adults between the ages 25-50 who had been hurt emotionally in the past by a significant event (divorce, fired from a job, infidelity of a spouse, injured by a reckless or drunk driver) experienced an average of a 40% reduction in depression and emotional pain after practicing a forgiveness exercise for just one week.

Another recent study at Hope College in Holland, Michigan, showed that merely holding the intention of forgiveness in mind has immediate effects on our health and energy levels. Researchers in this study attached sensors to a group of college-age students. They were asked to first relive a time in the past when they were hurt by someone. From there, they were directed to think about it in two different ways. One was to imagine getting revenge on the offender and punishing them. The other was to imagine forgiving the person and releasing the anger associated with the incident. Their findings were very interesting. The students' blood pressure and heart rate went up over 35% when they thought about acting out their revenge. When they considered forgiveness, they entered a state of 'coherence' where they enjoyed a relaxed heart rate and optimal blood pressure.

Coherence is somewhat of a spiritual state of being where brain waves, heart rate and breathing become aligned or 'in sync.' This creates expanded awareness and feelings of well-being. Chaos is the opposite of coherence. It occurs any time we're holding onto anger and it constricts the natural flow of healthy energy.

Additional health benefits from letting go of anger were reported in the *Journal of Epidemiology & Community Health*, November 2009. A study involving 2,755 people, with an average age of 41, were evaluated over a period of 10 years. Those who repressed anger and held resentments were found to be twice as likely to die of a heart attack compared to people in the study who were able to process and let go of negative feelings. The take-home message from the findings of this scientific study is: Forgiving others and releasing resentment can save your life, literally.

FORGIVENESS IS A CHOICE

Those who forgive are those who choose to forgive. There's nothing random or unintentional about it. It's an act of free will and a conscious decision to give up the desire to punish a person now, or in the future, for something that happened in the past. Forgiveness is not done out of weakness; it is an act of strength and courage.

Before we make the conscious decision to forgive someone, we must contemplate whether we're actually willing to do so. Ask yourself, "What do I gain by holding onto the idea of revenge?" Then, "What would I gain by letting go of the grievance?" While considering your answers, take note of the fact that the one who's most harmed by resentment is never the offender; it's you. Also, holding onto a grievance doesn't give you control over the offender; it gives them control over you. Oftentimes, the people we are unwilling to forgive don't even know we're upset with them, or have forgotten about the situation altogether. In some cases, there is reconciliation along with forgiveness, but in many cases there is not.

The price of unforgiveness is high and can include depression, a hot temper, anxiety, emotional pain that takes hold in the physical form (headaches, backaches, fatigue) and toxic amounts of stress. The benefits of forgiveness are many and include improved heart health, brighter energy, emotional well-being, decreased risk for disease and expanding spiritual awareness.

Another unfortunate thing about deeply held and suppressed anger towards someone is that it spills over and interferes with our relationships with everyone else. It can make us feel like we're always victims, and there is injustice in even the most insignificant daily incidents. For example, when we take it personally and lash out with anger as a car cuts in front of us in traffic. When someone reacts that way it's very often a sign that they are holding a pretty big charge of pent-up, inner anger. The more we dwell on hurtful events, grudges and vengeance, the more anger will take root in our minds and hearts. Before long, negative feelings can crowd out positive ones. Until the anger and bitterness are released, they will continue to leak poison into virtually all areas of your life, and can even destroy families, careers and friendships.

Offenders don't necessarily need to ask for forgiveness in order for you to grant it. In some cases, they might believe there is nothing for which they need to be forgiven. That's fine. We don't need to be concerned with how others perceive a situation as it really has no effect on us, unless we allow it to. Remember, when we hold a grudge, it doesn't punish the other person, it punishes us. And when we forgive, there's no guarantee the other person will change.

Oftentimes people limit their capacity to forgive by thinking that if they don't bring the offender to justice, nobody will. For me it's helpful to understand that I'm not judge and jury of the universe. I have absolute faith that the Source of life itself has everything under its control, and this being the case, it presides over all cases of injustice. When I forgive, I envision removing a pocket of negative energy from my awareness and turning it over to the Divine so it can be done away with. I don't picture delegating my grievance to a vengeful God with the expectation that it will punish the person for me.

Another factor which can contribute to a person's unwillingness to forgive arises from a common misunderstanding, which involves applying laws of the physical world to spiritual matters. In the world of matter, if I have a dollar in my hand and I give it to you, then you have one and I have none. Spiritual economics works differently. If I give compassion and forgiveness to you, my currency doesn't go down, it goes up. And if I resent you, my energy, or 'soul voltage' as I call it, diminishes. This also means that the cynic who can lure you into hating them is stealing your life currency and degradating your value. The more we love, the more we care, the more 'spiritually rich' we are. Literally and metaphorically we profit by giving forgiveness away.

Of course, in the nonphysical realm currency isn't counted in dollars, it's measured in what we might call vibrant frequency or light, which is the gold standard. John 1:7 (NIV) indicates that light and Divinity are one in the same. So in essence, practicing compassionate forgiveness may very well allow us to become more filled with the energy of light, or God as some would say.

Through the lens of the modern science of neurology, the brains of people who hold grudges and bitterness may show intense activity in the limbic system. This lower part of the brain is responsible for survival instincts, where resentment is held as fear. The consequences of living with fear include depression, irritability and self-loathing. Brain scans, which use SPECT (Single Photon Emission Computed Tomography) to look at which areas of the brain are most active, show when a person has a significantly cathartic experience through forgiveness, their brain can change significantly. The primal limbic system cools, allowing energy to flow more freely to the neocortex and right temporal lobe which are associated with decision making, compassion, intuition, as well as 'spiritual thinking' and behavior.

FORGIVE AND FORGET?

Forgiveness is something that happens inside of you. It doesn't mean you're saying what happened to cause a resentment wasn't wrong or that it didn't matter. What it means is that you're saying, "I choose to let go of this negative feeling towards the person whom I perceive has hurt me." After neutralizing the emotional charge behind the grievance by letting it go, you may very well file it away in your low-priority memory storage. It's not necessary to work on forgetting it altogether.

It's important to accept that we cannot change the past. What's done is done. Forgiveness helps us change the present and the future. It sets us free. But as long as we hold onto a grievance, we are chained to the past situation and the offender. This is paradoxical because in many cases people who have been harmed by someone want to be as far away from them as possible.

A result of practicing forgiveness is that it allows us to live more in the present moment. That's because as long as any part of our mind or consciousness is engaged with unresolved feelings from the past it will require us to expend valuable energy on it. And of course, to move forward and reach our transformation objectives, we really do have to harness all of our energy and apply it to what we're doing here and now.

HOW TO FORGIVE

True forgiveness involves becoming consciously aware of the resentment we're holding, then confessing it to at least one other person, while we allow ourselves to feel the emotion of it all. Talking it through with the unconditional support of another can help you process the memory and begin to get it out of your system. The next step is to directly communicate your forgiveness to the other person involved (by letter, phone or in person) in an empathic and sincere way. However, when directly sharing this would be potentially unsafe for you, and when reconciliation is not the objective, you can communicate through prayer or meditation how you are forgiving the person to your perception of a Higher Power or Source of life. From there, you must let it go once and for all.

Before you can practice forgiveness, you need to first look within yourself to identify a few incidents that you perceive were significantly harmful. It might be far back in the past or relatively recent. What I've discovered is that nearly everyone has been hurt by the actions or words of another. Perhaps you had a parent who criticized your every move or your partner had an affair. Maybe it's a time when you most remember being rejected, put down, treated unfairly, abandoned or even abused. It might be when someone harmed a member of your family or getting fired from a job. It might even be anger you hold toward yourself for a mistake you made. Or it could even be a resentment towards Divinity for what might have felt like an unfair loss of a loved one. When you have a moment, do a little introspection and see what comes to mind for you. Then grab a pen and a piece of paper and write down a few of the specific incidences. It helps to see it on paper, all out in front of you.

After that, take a few minutes and read over what you've written and briefly hold in mind each incident for a minute or two. Then I want you to rate the intensity of those feelings on a scale of 1-10. Maybe 1 is somebody cut in line in front of you at the grocery store, and 10 was the absolute worst thing that ever happened to you. Continue until you've rated all the incidences you've written down. Then, pick one of the most troubling ones and take note of the person you perceive was responsible for it. I call this incident 'The Big Hurt.'

START BY FORGIVING ONE

We're going to focus on one single event with this assignment. That's because truly forgiving one major offense and letting go of the resentment about it has been demonstrated to help people become forgiving in all aspects of their life. This was shown in a series of studies called 'The Stanford Forgiveness Project.' Researchers discovered that people who were taught to forgive one particular individual became much more forgiving in a broader, more generalized sense. They also developed greater overall control of their emotions, became less likely to get upset and were much less likely to feel hurt compared to those

111

who had not practiced a profound act of forgiveness. Many even found self-forgiveness in the process of forgiving another for something significant. Our full intention is to become consistently compassionate and generous with granting people forgiveness, and we can begin to embody this quality more than ever by completing the action step at the end of this chapter.

Once we've identified an especially strong resentment, we'll need to become clear about the feelings that arise when we bring our attention to the hurt. Then we try to identify just one way that holding onto the resentment benefits our well-being. Next we'll contemplate how our life might improve if we were able to completely eliminate the negative emotions that still simmer beneath the surface regarding this situation.

We'll also write a story about The Big Hurt. It can be a couple paragraphs or multiple pages. While doing this, we express our emotions, the hurt we felt and the anger that followed. We no longer have to hold onto them. For the process of forgiveness to be cleansing and purifying, it's necessary to feel, rather than deny, the hurtful emotions. Without doing that, saying "I forgive you" is superficial—it's just talk. The suppressed emotions will still be there.

In some cases, people have held onto their resentment for so long, it becomes a part of their identity and emotional structure. "Who will I be if I don't hate and seek revenge on this person or organization for ruining my life?" You'll be a healthier, happier version of you! And yes, it may require some time to get used to living free of the old pain, but it's a very good change no matter how you look at it. After you've written your story, I want you to then add a new ending to it: *"Even after all this, I unselfishly and courageously granted the offender complete forgiveness, out of the goodness of my heart. Through this act of grace and mercy, I have completely let go of the issue once and for all."*

You'll share your story with at least one other person and talk it through. Knowing this is your very last chance to focus on it, share your feelings openly and honestly. The act of true forgiveness may involve the release of a significant amount of bundled-up emotional energy. It's not uncommon at all for resentments to be washed away in tears as you heal. For others, it's gradual and they might need to do this work several times over a period of weeks in order to release the resentment 100%.

ACTION STEP:

After some introspection, these are three incidences and people which I've identified I hold some resentment towards:

Example:

1) Angry at my old boss for firing me from the job I enjoyed. (6)

2) Still upset at my ex-spouse for filing for divorce. (8)

3) Mad at myself for gaining so much weight. (7)

How I rate the emotional impact, on a scale of 1-10, of each of the grievances listed above is:

(Write down the ratings next to your list above.)

One way holding this resentment benefits my health is:

Example:

Can't think of one; maybe there aren't any.

Three feelings I would enjoy if I were able to completely eliminate this resentment from my mind and heart are:

Example:

1) Be lighter—a weight off my shoulders.

2) Relieved and more relaxed.

3) Renewed happiness and joyfulness.

Three ways my health and life would improve as a result of completely forgiving the offender and letting go of this resentment are:

Example:

1) Reduced risk of heart disease.

2) Less chance of suffering depression.

3) More energy and awareness to invest in healthy behaviors.

My Big Hurt story which expresses how I perceive the hurtful incident goes like this:

(In your own words, write out what you are feeling. It can be two paragraphs or several pages; it's up to you. Be sure to end your story with The Big Forgive declaration on the bottom of page 112.)

A nonjudgmental, unconditionally supportive person I can talk through my Big Hurt story with is:

Example:

Close friend, counselor, therapist, someone from the community.

Note: After you complete one act of forgiveness from start to finish, please consider setting yourself free from the other two resentments on your list. Simply follow the same action steps over again for each one.

CONCLUSION

Like Azim Khamisa, everyone has the power and ability to forgive others. And now is the time to rise up to a higher level of that potential. When you do, you'll enjoy greater health and well-being throughout every aspect of your life. Please remember as you work on this assignment that you will get out of it what you put into it. So reach into your heart and soul and give it all you've got. I promise you'll be happy you did.

114

9

Accepting Responsibility

Most every great transformation I've witnessed over the years was preceded by a dramatic increase of self-responsibility. The moment you truly decide to accept ownership of your health, happiness and life is the moment when everything begins to change. When you stop blaming others, give up the victim stories, and you accept responsibility, it's then and only then that you can harness your true power and ability to take control and make remarkable changes for the better.

Unfortunately, in our society today, we're conditioned to do pretty much just the opposite. Not happy? It's because of the people in my life. They're the ones making me miserable. Not healthy? It's the genetics I inherited. Darn ancestors! Crummy job? It's because of the government and how they screwed up the economy. Haven't been able to consistently eat right and exercise? That's because all the so-called experts make it so darn complicated and difficult for me; besides, I don't have time because everyone else expects me to take care of them first.

 115

Get the idea?

These kinds of excuses can seem very real and valid when we mistakenly believe that someone else is responsible for how we're doing. When we do that, we literally give away our power to change. And as much as we might want to lose weight, feel more energetic and succeed, we'll experience frustration, disappointment, and before long, we'll quit. And then of course, we'll blame someone else for it.

The good news is, we can each take that power back anytime we choose to. To do that, we swallow our pride, move beyond the defense tactics of our egoic self, and place the blame where it belongs: on the person we see when we stand in front of the mirror. Yes, I know it seems more 'comfortable' to imagine that the things we don't like about our bodies, our work and our relationships are someone else's fault. But that's a trap that will imprison us until we face the real facts.

Accepting responsibility means taking control of the things you can and letting go of everything else. This is a very important point. What other people do, what they say, what they think… that's their responsibility, not ours. We have no control over anything that happens in the world except what we do, what we say, what we think, and how we choose to respond to the events of this day.

It's unfortunate to see that so many folks waste such vast quantities of valuable energy worrying about, gossiping about and complaining about things that are beyond their control. When we do that, we're not solving anything, we're not transforming anything, we're not helping ourselves or anyone else. The only thing blaming and complaining really does is attract other people who do the same.

One of the telltale signs that we've given our power away (either knowingly or unknowingly) is by the excuses we make. By their nature, excuses deny our responsibility. Those who've taken control of the things they can in their life choose to share the reasons why things are the way they are, even when those reasons might not always make them look good. (Excuse: The dog ate my homework. Reason: My homework's not done because I chose to watch TV instead of doing it.)

RESULTS ARE NOT OUR RESPONSIBILITY

Those of us who enjoy and understand the power of setting goals and doing the work to achieve them often make a common mistake. It's one that can cause our confidence to crumble and zap our energy and motivation. The error is assuming that we have control over results. The fact is, we don't.

Consider this example: We plant seeds in the soil of a flower garden. We can control how much water the garden gets, how much the soil is nourished, and we can clear away weeds and obstructions so that the sunlight gets in. But, and this is a big but, we can't make the flowers grow. That's beyond our control and therefore not our responsibility. Whatever the power is that created life to begin with is in charge of such matters. We can take responsibility for creating the right conditions in the garden, but when the flower blooms, it's an illusion to believe that we made it happen.

The same is true with our bodies and lives. We're responsible for creating the right conditions; we're not in control of the results. When we come to truly accept and understand this, we again experience a powerful shift in our mindset. At that point, our specific goals for the future become guideposts that show us which actions we need to take in order to create the right conditions for transformation to occur.

Again, I want to emphasize that whatever the intelligent, creative energy is that gave us life in the first place (however you want to see that) is what's responsible for any healing and renewal of our bodies, minds and emotions. That force is always there, trying to do its job—trying to restore healthy balance. What stands in its way is typically the fact that our thoughts and actions have been creating the wrong conditions.

117

Knowing this, it becomes clear that in order to feel a sense of accomplishment, confidence, and positive energy, we need to measure our success not by results but whether we honored our responsibility and took control of the things that are within our reach. For example, we can control whether we exercise today or not; whether we eat healthy today or not; whether we follow through and complete our weekly action steps or not.

When we do those things, we've done all we can. From there it's important to surrender the rest. We actually must let go of any attachment to the outcome and have faith that whatever's meant to happen from there will happen. Not only does that help us enjoy peace of mind and fulfillment, but according to experts in the manifesting process, letting go is essential for the creative culmination of what was set in motion.

HOW DO WE KNOW IF WE'VE TRULY LET GO?

A sure sign that we haven't let go is that we ruminate and fuss—we question ourselves and the method. In doing so, we send out a conflicted, untrusting energy frequency which not only negatively affects our emotional health, but again, according to many wise and thoughtful teachers, interferes with the fulfillment and receiving of the best possible outcome. Those who truly get that all they can do is the best they can do at the things that are within their control enjoy better results and have a more confident mindset too.

NO EXCUSES

When we make a resolute decision to accept responsibility for our own health and happiness we are, in effect, becoming a 'no-excuses person.' This is not an action, it's a mental shift. In this stage, we're conditioning our minds, or rather un-conditioning them, to reflect the reality that we're in charge of our own well-being. In this stage, you might wake up and you really don't feel like doing your workout. Rather than making an excuse that you don't have time today, we learn to see in that moment we simply don't want to do it.

That's fine. The fact is, I rarely feel like exercising when I get up in the morning but rather than making an excuse, I say, "I'm choosing to take control of my health today and so I'm going to exercise even though right now, I don't really want to."

I know from firsthand experience that we can transform our thought patterns and eliminate excuses. To do that, we accept responsibility for what we choose. If we sit on the sofa all weekend and veg out, rather than thinking, "I'm too tired to do anything because my boss gave me so much work to do this week," we should instead say, "I'm choosing to veg out." The truth is, there really isn't anything preventing us from getting up and being active except the choice we make. And since our choices are within our control, they're our responsibility also. Realizing this leads to a crucial mental shift that prepares us to resume complete control of our lives.

SELFISH VS. SELF-RESPONSIBILITY

Oftentimes people mistakenly believe that by accepting responsibility to take care of their own health and happiness, they're somehow being selfish. And no mature, conscious person wants to be called "selfish." This is yet another obstacle we need to overcome in order to reclaim sovereignty in our own lives. The fact is, we are being self-responsible when we prioritize, each day, doing what we need to in order to recover and renew our physical, mental and emotional well-being. That means we must choose to make time for exercise, eating healthy meals, rest, recovery and sleep. We must choose to create at least some quiet time for self-reflection and to clear and calm the mind.

We must also choose to make time for doing things which we enjoy and that bring us happiness. These can be very simple things, for example: taking an evening walk at sunset; listening to your favorite music; getting out to enjoy your favorite hobby on a weekend. Although this all sounds simple, if we perceive them as being selfish, we'll resist and put them off.

119

Remember, you and only you are responsible for your well-being. I can offer a proven plan—one that's worked for thousands of people from all walks of life—but only you can follow through and do it. If you need to reach out for help from a counselor or doctor, that too is your responsibility. Following through with doctor's orders is not something anyone is going to do for us. As much as we might want to believe that our well-being is the health-care system's responsibility, again, it's not. Other people can encourage and support you and you can significantly benefit from that, but even the most helpful people in the world can't do the transformation work and action steps for you.

Knowing what we have control over and accepting responsibility for it is remarkably empowering. When you reach that point, you really can become the pilot of your life and make it better and brighter than it's ever been. When you do, you'll have more life energy and strength to unselfishly give to others.

ACTION STEP:

Three specific excuses that I've used multiple times to avoid taking responsibility for my own condition are:

Example:

1) *I haven't been consistently eating healthy because my spouse still insists on eating junk food.*

2) *I haven't been getting in my workouts because I don't have time.*

3) *Everyone in my family tree has suffered from overweight and obesity; that's why I can't lose weight.*

Three things I'm taking control of, starting today, are:

Example:

1) *My health.*

2) *My time.*

3) *My mindset.*

Three actions I'll take this week to demonstrate that I'm accepting responsibility for the things I've written above are:

Example:

1) *My health: I'm no longer going to eat junk food; instead, I'm going to make the conscious decision to eat healthy foods.*

2) *My time: Plan my days in advance and choose to set firm boundaries around the time I need to take care of myself.*

3) *My mindset: Choose to see setbacks and adversity as opportunities to learn, grow and improve.*

Three things I realize are beyond my control which I surrender are:

Example:

1) *I have no control of how others respond to my decision to transform my life.*

2) *I surrender my attachment to outcomes and the results which come from the work I do.*

3) *I'm not responsible for the actual healing process; I have faith that when I give these assignments my all that the Source of life itself will do the rest.*

CONCLUSION

We must each give up blaming others for our lack of fulfillment, well-being and success. Instead, we can accept full responsibility for the condition of our lives. When we do, then and only then will we tap into our fullest potential and ability to change. As we continue on, we give up our excuses and fully realize it's up to us to consciously choose how we respond and what we do in any given moment. By taking responsibility for those things that are within your control, and surrendering everything else, you will discover renewed energy, power and peace of mind.

10

The Positive Mindset

Unlike the physical body, the mind is very fluid and it can take on a new form in an instant. We can be confident, believing in our ability one moment, doubtful and uncertain the next. This can be especially true when taking on something new and challenging like this transformation process.

In order for us to successfully reach our goals with this work, we must know how to set and reset the mind in a positive direction. Here are 4 tried-and-true techniques to transform your mindset in minutes:

1) TAKE ACTION

The longer we procrastinate and avoid taking action, the tighter the grip of fearful and apprehensive thoughts becomes. There's a surefire way to put an end to that. It's to get up, get moving, and as Nike says, *just do it*.

Whether it's taking on a challenging project that you've been putting off, getting in your daily workout or taking a before photo and sharing it with at least one other person, the method works the same. The moment you start

123

taking action, thoughts of uncertainty and feelings of anxiety immediately begin to fade. In their place you'll find a more positive, can-do state of mind. Each and every day will be that way, as long as you keep moving. Again, I can't emphasize enough that so very often the solution to what seems like it's keeping a person stuck is nothing more and nothing less than all-out ACTION. This is something Albert Einstein noticed too. He said that when it comes to physics, nothing happens until something moves. I think the same is true for us. So add more action—more motion—to your life today.

2) FOCUS ON WHAT'S WORKING

We always tend to get more of what we focus on in life. It's true. This means it's vitally important to be mindful of where our attention is. If we have a habitual pattern of looking at what's not working, according to this tenet, we'll be getting more of that—more of what's not working.

On the other hand, if we mindfully choose to focus on what's working, we'll be cultivating more successful results. That's because what a human being directs its attention towards receives a flow of consciousness or thought energy. Think of it as light; wherever it shines in a garden there will be growth. This is true for flowers and weeds. Very often, people's mindsets can become affixed or stuck in a certain direction. When that happens, no matter how much they want to transform, they won't be able to because they continue to see the same things day after day and they continue to manifest the same results in their lives that they have before. It reminds me of a cartoon where there's a character standing outdoors, the entire bright blue sky is filled with sunshine except there's a small dark cloud over just that one person. And the micro-storm follows them wherever they go.

Please remember that energy flows where your attention goes. So focus on what you love, what makes you smile, and what makes you feel healthy, and alive! In doing so, you'll soon have even more to be happy about.

3) THE POWER OF WORDS

The words we say to others *and ourselves* directly influence our mindset, health, and actions for better or worse every single day. Positive language has been demonstrated to improve scores on aptitude tests, boost physical performance, and even strengthen the immune system. And negative talk can do just the opposite.

I remember when someone exclaimed, "Good heavens! You can't lift that much weight. It's going to crush you!" as I held 385 lbs over my chest in a state powerlifting contest when I was back in my 20s. Sure enough, that barbell came down at record speed and just laid there on my rib cage.

Despite having lifted this much weight and more dozens of times in my training, at that moment, it felt like my elbows and shoulders just gave out. On the other hand, in the gym, I had a very confident and bright training partner who was a masterful encourager. He was always telling me what I could do and how much strength I had within me. Those two examples have stuck with me all these years and have taught me firsthand, the power of words.

Scientific studies also show that language makes a difference. For example, the National Institute of Child Health and Human Development reported survey findings in the *Journal of the American Medical Association* (April 25, 2001) explaining that there is widespread use of 'bullying' and harmful language directed towards children throughout most U.S. schools. And another report titled *Implications for Prevention of School Attacks in the U.S.* says that attackers in school shootings felt bullied, persecuted, and verbally injured by others prior to the attack.

Another study at Stanford University, conducted July 1999 through June 2003, demonstrated that eliminating kids' exposure to harsh language they had been hearing on TV and video games, produced a 50% decrease in the kids' verbal aggression and a 40% decrease in physical aggression. In a separate study, it was demonstrated that when test subjects were addressed with kind, caring, and affirmative words, the strength of their immune systems went up significantly within a matter of minutes and they remained elevated for up to two hours.

The power of words can hurt or help people of all ages. *The Journal of the American Geriatrics Society* (November 22,1999) reported that empowering words and positive talk significantly improve the state of mind of the elderly, resulting in improved function and well-being.

Most all of us have felt the power of words working in our own lives on many occasions. And in the case of transformation, a process that involves making numerous challenging changes, it's imperative that you have some exposure to positive, affirmative and uplifting talk. This is another place where inspired, supportive friends from your communities can be a big help. When they see the best in you, recognize your potential, and remind you of the positive steps you're taking to improve your health and life, it can lift your energy, courage, and motivation as well as strengthen your resilience.

Keep in mind also that the words you use in your own self-talk can either be deflating and demoralizing or nurturing and reinforcing. It's vitally important that you recognize critical self-talk fast and replace it with something positive. Many of the people that I help through the transformation process start out by essentially being their own worst enemy—their own bully—and by the time we complete the process, they've transformed that negative into a positive. Their self-talk becomes a source of energy, encouragement, and self esteem.

To harness the positive power of words and put them to work in your own life, you simply start by being more mindful about what you're saying, how you're saying it, and what effect it's having on others as well as yourself. Then speak often of inspiration, love, gratitude, health and healing, and how you're transforming, improving, and making good progress. The more you do, the more you will.

126

4) ENVISIONING SUCCESS

Another effective way to shift your mindset is to envision a successful out-come. Many people who do well with their personal transformation make a daily practice to see, in their mind, where they're going before they get there. They envision, with crystal clarity, what their renewed body and improved life will be like. For many this becomes a very powerful practice.

This past year I've helped a dozen people who began their journey 60 to 100 lbs overweight. We worked on creating a clear mental image of their bod-ies as lean and strong before every exercise session.

Within a few weeks most of them began to identify with the future vision of themselves more than who they saw in their before photos. I also teach them to begin thinking and behaving like the version of themselves they see on the horizon. What would the new you do in a given situation, blow off today's workout or find a way to get it done? Would the new version of yourself pro-crastinate and waste time, or make the most of every minute, of every day? Shifting your mindset so you begin to think like the person you're envisioning is a powerful change because thoughts, intentions and ideas always occur first. The physical manifestation is a secondary phenomenon.

Unfortunately, sometimes people can significantly change the way they look on the outside by losing weight or building muscle but they stay very much the same on the inside. They still have the same patterns of thinking, beliefs, and perspectives. In cases like these the recidivism rate is very nearly 100%. I don't want this to happen to you, which is why I highly encourage changing your mindset as a fundamental step to sustainable results.

Please consider making a few minutes of quiet time each day to sit in still-ness and hold an image in mind of how you want to be, how you want to look, how you want to feel. When you do, you may very well be surprised with how rapidly that inner vision becomes your external reality.

ACTION STEP:

Empowering words and phrases that I will utilize in my daily communication with others and myself include:

Example:

Inspired, energized, strong, happy, kind, grateful, positive, healthy, successful, focused, bright, blessed, and transforming.

A description of the future self I envision is:

Example:

I feel inspired and energetic. I make mindful decisions which support and nurture my well-being. I am kind and caring towards all. My body looks healthy and strong. I am smiling and happy.

Three empowering, healthy thoughts which are aligned with my transformation objectives are:

Example:

1) *I feel healthy, positive and strong.*
2) *The transformation methods which have worked for so many others will work for me too.*
3) *I do have the time to take care of myself and improve my life.*

CONCLUSION

To transform your mindset, start by taking action and getting the things done that you need to do to achieve your goals. Then direct your attention towards what's working and away from what's not. Your mindset will be further strengthened and renewed by utilizing positive and affirmative words with others and yourself. And envisioning the way you want to look, feel and think in the future will absolutely help you get there. When you put it all together you'll have the kind of mindset that makes anything possible!

128

11

Releasing Concealments

Transformation is a process of making healthy changes both inside and out. To do this we focus on improving ourselves in all of these areas:

1) PHYSICALLY

Regular exercise and eating the right nutrition allow the body to let go of unhealthy pounds while strengthening muscles, improving metabolism, lifting energy, and even enhancing our ability to think clearly. This foundational aspect must be in place in order to optimally support our inner-transformation. Bringing our physical form into healthy balance facilitates the flow of higher vibrational energies. It also strengthens our grounding and stability.

2) MENTALLY

Becoming clear about where we are and where we want to be, then channeling that awareness into specific, objectively verifiable goals, with timelines and deadlines, give us a healthy mental focus. When we follow that up with consistently planning our healthy days ahead of time and comparing our actual behavior to what we intended, it allows the mind the kind of feedback it needs to learn and sharpen its focus. Seeing our progress rather than our lack of perfection gives us a dependable source of self-confidence. And working to achieve a consistently positive mindset gives us a big advantage that's hard to be successful without.

3) SPIRITUALLY

Helping others, with no expectations of receiving something in return, and unconditionally supporting, encouraging, and caring for those in our various communities, enlivens our spiritual well-being. In this context, our 'spiritual nature' is the non-individual aspect of each of us; it's where we're all connected as one borderless, worldwide family.

Any time we authentically look beyond our own self-interests and act in a way that benefits the greater good, we are aligning with and honoring the spiritual aspect of us, individually and collectively. As we continue to give what we have to give (sharing our experience, our life lessons, our talents and even resources) we are certain to continue our spiritual growth.

4) EMOTIONALLY

Letting go of repressed anger and resentments through courageous and bold acts of forgiveness helps us begin to heal emotionally. This is vitally important because in a very real way, our bodies and lives tend to reflect our inner-emotional condition. Yes, we can lose weight and even build stronger muscles without improving our emotional well-being. But even when people's bodies begin to look better, it doesn't always mean they're happier or more joyful inside. And as such, the initial physical improvements may not be sustained for very long. The better approach is to cultivate emotional health throughout the process. And that's what we'll be doing now by releasing concealments from the shadows into the light.

WHAT ARE CONCEALMENTS?

Concealments are those things we don't want to deal with, admit or confront, which have been repressed (stuffed away beneath our conscious awareness). They include fears, insecurities, negative thoughts, traumatic memories, embarrassing things we've done that we feel guilty and shameful about.

On the surface, it makes sense to hide those things away, especially in today's society where we're often taught that admittance of any kind of mistake, indiscretion or personal struggle is a sign of 'weakness' and that it makes us inherently 'bad' in some way. Along with that, I find that there's generally a widespread misunderstanding that concealments somehow go away if we suppress and avoid them long enough. Unfortunately, that's not the case. They're like a debt owed to the IRS... sooner or later you're going to have to pay up.

You see, anything you suppress and conceal is stored in the body, on a cellular level, where it eventually becomes a toxin. Scientific studies have demonstrated rather clearly that these unprocessed emotions and feelings lead to significantly higher rates of depression, anxiety, weakened immune system, stress, compulsive eating (and the weight gain that comes with it), higher rates of drug and alcohol abuse, as well as a significantly greater risk of dying of a heart attack.

Not only that, concealments can interfere with our ability to experience our true emotions. It's almost like they block the river which contains the natural flow of our feelings, and that causes them to build up a reservoir of difficult as well as joyful and beautiful experiences. This continues until they're properly resolved and released.

HOW DO WE RELEASE CONCEALMENTS?

Fortunately, releasing concealments is not at all complicated; in fact, it's pretty simple. (I said simple, not easy.) And the benefits are remarkable. Letting go of unhealthy repressions allows us to live our lives in greater truth and authenticity, free from the anxiety and fear of being 'found out.' It breaks the dam and lets the natural flow of our emotional energy and current. This in turn opens the heart, allows our consciousness to expand, and makes us feel more connected to ourselves, others and the Source of life itself. Our relationships become more stable and loving, our health improves in every way, intuition and perception become more fine-tuned and it also seems to open the doors to new opportunities.

This kind of emotional healing has been included in the wisdom traditions and practices of cultures around the world, dating back several thousand years. It's a cornerstone to religions including Christianity, Judaism, Hinduism, Buddhism and Sufism. Native American Indians and Aboriginal tribes also have a long history of healing rituals which include confession and speaking one's truth. Modern psychology and addiction recovery programs also place a strong emphasis on revealing secrets in order to restore mental and emotional health.

The power of this practice is activated when we do these three things:

1) Identify concealments through quiet introspection. We look for feelings and memories that we've avoided dealing with in the past and we keep looking, right on up to the present. We're especially looking for things that make us feel guilt, shame, anxiety, even fear when we bring them to mind.

2) Confront concealments and acknowledge them by writing them down on a sheet of paper where they can be acknowledged and brought out into the light of our full awareness.

3) Confess them to another person. This can be a nonjudgmental friend, family member, counselor, priest, rabbi, spiritual leader, or a trusted member of the community.

That's how simple and basic this healing exercise is. And yes I know, I'd rather have a cavity drilled and filled without Novocain too, rather than do this assignment. But that's what makes it so powerful. We grow by confronting things that we are apprehensive about or uncomfortable with. When we move away from what we fear, it becomes a bigger and more dominant force in our life; but when we move towards it, it becomes smaller and smaller until it has little or no effect on us. And this is precisely what releasing conceal-ments is all about.

You see, the reason these repressions become harmful to our health is because at some level we're always afraid that our secret will get out and we'll be rejected for it. The centers of the brain responsible for our 'survival behavior' interpret this anxiety as a threat to our existence and send out the same sort of fight or flight neurochemicals and reflexes that it would if we confronted a bear while hiking through the woods. The difference being that after we safely escaped from the bear and that danger, our defense systems would relax and return to normal.

With hidden concealments, to some degree we're always on guard, espe-cially around intuitive, open people whose awareness is not easily fooled. It takes a lot of energy to maintain the defense system that keeps your conceal-ments hidden from others as well as from your own conscious mind. This can be so draining that we isolate and disconnect more and more because it simply takes too much effort to keep that shield up when we're out in public and around other people for any considerable amount of time.

By doing the action steps at the end of this chapter you're going to get your energy back. You're also going to feel lighter by releasing concealments because they weigh on your heart and mind the whole time you're carrying them around.

It can be a bit of a challenge to identify some concealments because it's been so long since we stuffed them away that we might have forgotten them altogether. What helps is to identify situations in the present which activate an emotional charge, perhaps causing frustration, blame, anger or anxiety, and then ask yourself if you've experienced that same kind of feeling at any time in the past, and see what comes to mind.

Oftentimes, the things we feel guilty and embarrassed about which have been suppressed will seep into our everyday interpretation of life. For example, if we've done something that we knew wasn't right, but chose not to deal with it at the time and instead stuffed it away, this can cause us to subconsciously see ourselves as a bad person. But our egoic self, especially when it's the dominant force in our personality, simply 'can't handle the truth' and so it projects what it doesn't want to see onto others.

For the experiencer, this can make the world seem like it's filled with untrustworthy and 'bad' people. On the other hand, someone whose conscience is clear and their emotions healthy, who feels good about themselves, may approach those same people with care, kindness, and appreciation for their fundamental qualities. So in this way, releasing concealments can help change the way we see the world and also how we respond to it.

When we're probing and seeking to identify things that we might have suppressed and concealed, that's the time to be very thoughtful. Sometimes it will take a good amount of work to identify issues but other times things will come to mind right away. These can be instances where we did something that was against our true character that hurt ourselves, or others, a little or perhaps a lot. In these instances we may very well recognize the need to ask for forgiveness from someone else after we've released the concealment. (We'll explore how best to do that in the next chapter.)

Once we've thoughtfully identified some unhealthy concealments it's important not to over-think things from there. In order to process these things it's essential that we feel them (rather than just intellectually grasp them). Healing occurs by experiencing the *emotions* we've been avoiding—the embarrassment, shame, guilt, sadness, concern and such.

We don't have to feel them for a long time or ruminate in them. My approach is to feel them fast and then let 'em go. Repressions can be released at the cellular level through this approach. This is something that a series of

134

scientific studies by James Pennebaker, a professor of psychology at Southern Methodist University, demonstrated. In these studies it was discovered that we must begin with earnest 'self reflective' thought (soul searching) to identify the issues and then follow that with honest and emotional expression.

Pennebaker's scientific studies also show that the health benefits of 'confession' tend to be proportional to the seriousness of the matter disclosed and also the most positive results occur when someone really opens up and shares their true innermost feelings. So basically, the more you put into it, the more you get out of it (we can say the same thing about virtually all the action steps in this book).

From my experience, the most dreadful aspect of releasing concealments is 'confessing them to another person.' But there's just no getting around it. I had my first major experience with this kind of work during a very intense emotional renewal retreat I signed up for as I entered my 40s some years ago. Through that experience I discovered that what I had made such a big deal about in my mind, which I carried and concealed for years, is not really a big deal at all in the grand scheme of things.

When I did the work to identify some issues that I felt bad about, and then when I confronted and acknowledged them to myself, I got stuck at that point for a few days. You see, the egoic mind (that aspect of ourselves that attempts to defend and protect us in the external world) says loud and clear, "No way is this stuff getting out; not while I'm in charge!" And that's what's so great about moving forward with the confession part; it immediately breaks the stranglehold the egoic nature can have on our minds.

The instant we begin to share these concealments with another, the ego is significantly diminished and we go through a transformation of sorts which makes us much more humble but yet more empowered at the same time. From a neurological standpoint what happens is the limbic system (responsible for fear and survival instincts) begins to 'relax' allowing energy to flow to other parts of the brain which give rise to greater compassion, empathy, creativity, and even more clear thinking.

The first time I went through this I really had to grit it out as I spoke about the mistakes I made. I sat with a mentor and kept my eyes on my written notes as I began.

"When I was in my early 20s, I used anabolic steroids, which I purchased illegally on the black market." I paused, took a deep breath, then continued.

"Another unhealthy mistake I made that I feel foolish about, is taking a multi-summer, hedonistic world tour in my 30s. I and a couple of friends went from Los Angeles, to Las Vegas, to Cabo, to Denver, New York, London, Paris, Athens and Hong Kong as we drank ridiculous amounts of tequila and beer and partied for nights in a row at clubs, cabarets and concerts. I did this on my own free will and understood it was not intelligent or healthy."

Again, I'd have to pause as my hands were trembling and my voice shaking from the overwhelming feelings of embarrassment and remorse.

I went on to confess everything from the time I went out with my first girl-friend's sister, to the time right before the retreat when I got into an argument with a family member. I just got every mistake I felt bad about out in the open.

After I finished, I sheepishly looked up at the person who was helping me with the exercise and I'll never forget it. He smiled just a bit, not like it was funny but rather that he was happy for me. He then said, "Is that it?" I was expecting at least an "Eegads!" Make no mistake, the stuff on a list like this never makes it to people's eHarmony profile page; it's too embarrassing. But to a nonjudgmental person who's also been through the emotional healing process, our concealments, which we have spent so much energy trying to suppress, are accepted and understood as aspects of the human experience.

The mentor who I was working with at the time explained, "Power comes from telling the truth. That's all there is to it." Then he looked at me and smiled, "I'll bet you wish you had done that a lot sooner, huh?" My answer was an affirmative, "Yes!" It really isn't something to put off or feel overly intimidated by. I'll tell you something for sure, ever since that first experience I've been much more accepting, understanding, and better able to empathize while also being less judgmental with others because it becomes stark ravingly clear that I'm not perfect either. When you 'get' this experientially it really can shift your perspective. It's helped me realize that everybody pretty much does the best they can with what they have to work with at any given point.

Yes, most all of us have effed up mightily somewhere along the road of life (watch out for people who say they haven't). The sooner and more often we come clean about it, the faster we can put it behind us and move on. I also know that we can all learn and change and grow if we truly want to. We don't have to keep making the same mistakes over and over again. But for us to improve and go forward we have to get around the defense systems, the denial and avoidance, and we must admit to ourselves and another where we're at and what is really, truly going on with us.

Now what I do is 'clear the deck' so to speak by identifying, confronting and confessing three specific things I feel uncomfortable about each and every week. Once you get this process started, things from the past tend to come to mind on a pretty continual basis which allows us to chip away at that unhealthy inner weight in a very thorough way. I also try to clear out any recent feelings that aren't sitting quite right with me. I figure once we get the closet close to clean there's no sense continuing to let it clutter up again.

The process of releasing concealments creates tremendous peace of mind and allows me to sleep easy at night, free from worry and regret. I have noticed though that I can't even throw a gum wrapper out on the street without thinking twice because I know I'd feel guilty about it and have to confess it later. And that's a good thing; it might just be the most profoundly positive effect of all because it can allow us all to recognize, prior to the moment of decision, how a certain action or behavior is going to make us feel.

137

ACTION STEP:

Through mindful introspection (soul searching) I've identified these three specific concealments as ones that are weighing on me and which I would like to be free of:

Example:

1) Used anabolic steroids in my 20s.

2) Partied way too much in my 30s.

3) Argued with a family member.

A nonjudgmental, unconditionally caring person whom I can share my truth with is:

Example:

A close friend, family member, counselor, spiritual leader, mentor, partner from the transformation community.

A specific time and place where I plan to release my concealments by sharing them with another person is:

Example:

Sunday morning with my pastor at church or a meeting with a friend.

Three ways I'll benefit when I identify, confront and confess my unhealthy concealments are:

Example:

1) I'll be able to sleep more soundly at night.

2) I will feel more comfortable being my authentic self instead of feel-ing anxious around others.

3) I'll experience less inner-conflict and stress which will make it eas-ier for me to not overeat or engage in unhealthy habits.

CONCLUSION

Releasing concealments is an essential step in the true transformation process. It frees the mind, lightens the heart and energizes the body. You can experience all those benefits when you identify uncomfortable feelings that you might be avoiding, boldly confront and acknowledge them in writing, and then courageously confess them to at least one other person who cares about your well-being, and who is nonjudgmental with their support. This action step is not easy, but it is so very much worth the effort. When you get it done, you'll discover renewed emotional health, happiness, and humility.

139

12

Making It Right

Having had the opportunity to invest the better part of the last decade towards exploring and learning about the healing and spiritual traditions of modern and ancient cultures from around the world, a few things have become very clear. One of which is that at the heart of the world's great teachings is a remarkably powerful, yet relatively simple set of instructions—a sort of 'Owner's Guide'—which spells out how to renew the health of our minds and emotions.

Examples include practices such as forgiveness, confession (releasing concealments), prayer (intention) and being of service to others. Through your action steps thus far, you've gained some powerful and practical knowledge about each one of these practices.

Those who've been doing the action steps wholeheartedly have also gained valuable firsthand experience in these areas as well. And now, we add another universal healing principle to our method with this chapter, Making it Right.

Making it right allows us to heal and resolve interpersonal conflict that very typically weighs on our hearts and minds, producing feelings of guilt and remorse. In religious and spiritual teachings this is called atonement ('at-one' or 'one-ment'). This is also referred to as making amends (mend-ing). It's a return to harmony and unity between people and one's Source of life.

In the Jewish tradition, the holiest day of the year, Yom Kippur, is specifically known as the 'Day of Atonement.' This holiday follows 10 days after Rosh Hashanah which is celebrated as the time of new beginnings, a new year. During the days between Rosh Hashanah and Yom Kippur people are encouraged to focus on deeds of charity, repentance (remorse and change), forgiving others and atonement (apologizing and asking for forgiveness).

I've gained a tremendous appreciation for the value of this tradition and its healing potential. Even from a Western scientific and psychological perspective, dedicating the first 10 days of a new year to clearing the mind of negative thoughts and hurtful emotions is a wonderful prescription; in fact, I believe that we should do these things throughout the year as well.

In the Orthodox Christian tradition, the reconciliation between man and Divinity is made possible by the sacrificial death and blood of Jesus Christ (taken literally or metaphorically). Atonement between individuals is considered very important—asking for and granting forgiveness is somewhat of a spiritual duty.

Buddhism has no specific practice of atonement with God (as it doesn't recognize a Supreme Being); however, it does teach the importance of mending division between people. When there's bitterness between one person and another, it is thought to lead to the development of negative and harmful emotions by way of their *karmic effect*.

The 12-step movement considers making amends essential for addiction recovery. It's widely believed that inner conflict is a causative factor for drug and alcohol abuse. But you don't have to be struggling with a dangerously bad habit to benefit from this practice. In fact, steps 8 and 9, which deal with amends in the AA model, weren't originally intended for that application at all. The basis of 12-step work was adapted from the teachings of a Lutheran pastor named Dr. Frank Buchman. He became popular in Europe and America in the 1920s and 30s and his followers were called collectively, the 'Oxford Group.'

Buchman taught that all change happens within the individual before it manifests outwardly. All people will make errors and all people can change, Buchman emphasized. The Oxford Group practiced openly and honestly sharing their past mistakes and troubles with one another and also worked at mending and renewing peace with anyone they had harmed through their words or actions in the course of their lives.

Modern psychology considers rifts between people, especially when they lead to feelings of guilt and self-reproach, as issues that can adversely affect mental health. Recent discoveries in neurology (science and study of the brain) show that there may indeed be positive effects on brain health when we process and let go of hurt feelings through practices like atonement.

In a recent study published in the *Journal of Psychosomatic Medicine*, research scientists discovered that those who work through feelings of guilt by making amends notice a significant increase in the strength of their immune system which makes them more resistant to infections, colds and dozens of chronic diseases.

Despite atonement's rich history in wisdom teachings throughout the ages, it's an all-but-forgotten and ignored tradition in today's modern world. But as I see it, with depression, stress and other forms of mental and emotional disease at an all-time high, now is a good time to get back to basics and begin living by these tried-and-true principles. To do so you don't need to adopt any new beliefs and you don't even have to be religious. This is something that can help virtually anyone enjoy greater health and happiness.

HOW TO MAKE AMENDS THE RIGHT WAY

What's worked really well for me and what I teach people I'm guiding through the transformation process are the '7 Keys to Making it Right.' This method can bring about a very deep healing experience for both you and the person who may have been offended or hurt by your actions.

1) The first key is to identify a specific incident that, upon reflection, you realize might have hurt someone else. Look for something that you feel significantly remorseful about and wish you wouldn't have done, or would have done differently.

2) Write down your thoughts and feelings about the incident to get them out in the open. Describe what happened and how it makes you feel when you consider it. How might it have made the other person feel? What can you do to make it right?

3) Talk it through with someone who you know supports you unconditionally and cares about your well-being. Share how you feel about it and how you plan to make it right.

4) When possible and appropriate, contact the person who might have been offended by your words and actions. You can do this by writing a thoughtful letter or email, making a phone call or meeting with the person face to face.

5) Offer a sincere, heartfelt apology, accept responsibility and admit to any wrongdoings. Also show your remorse and empathy.

6) The sixth key is offering to do something to make it right. Include specific detail about the changes you'll make so as to not let it happen again.

7) Forgive yourself. We all make mistakes on our journey through life. By extending a sincere apology and offering to make it right, you can feel really good about yourself because not a lot of people in today's world are being so considerate. Take a deep breath and let go of any guilt and self-blame on the exhale. Smile and allow yourself to feel grateful for the lessons learned.

IT WORKS OFTEN, BUT NOT ALWAYS

Even when we do our best to apologize and make it right, there's no guaranteeing the other person will forgive us. And so we accept, from the outset, that all we can do is the best we can do and the outcome is beyond our control. As such, we must not be attached to it.

What I've discovered is that most often people respond very well to sincere apologies and are willing to let it go, especially if they can feel your true remorse. But every once in a while we're bound to encounter someone who just isn't ready to give up the grievance. A lot of this has to do with where they are on the path and what they're personally going through.

This happens sometimes and it does no good to be despondent about it. You can simply mention that your offer of atonement is open and if at any time in the future they might be so kind as to accept your apology and forgive you, it would mean a lot.

Occasionally, you might find that when making amends to someone they feel no apology is necessary. Because we all interpret and respond to the things people do and say in a subjective way, what might seem like it was harmful on our part doesn't always affect others adversely. I can think of a few occasions where I felt remorseful about something I did or said but then came to discover the person I felt I might have offended didn't consider it a big deal at all. In cases like that, I've discovered it still helps to share my feelings about the situation as well as what I learned from it.

Here's something else I want you to keep in mind: We won't always know who might hold a resentment or grudge towards us. Again, because we all experience the things people do and say somewhat differently, what might have seemed incidental to us may have offended another. If you can sense that someone may be feeling resentful towards you it can be helpful to ask the person about it and be open to hearing what they have to say.

ACTION STEP:

An incident I've identified from my distant or recent past where, upon reflection, I feel responsible for causing someone to become hurt or offended can be described as:

Example:

Argued with a family member over a misunderstanding.

A description of my thoughts and feelings about what happened and what the other person might have experienced goes like this:

Example:

I feel remorseful and very sorry about the incident. I feel that I hurt someone's feelings.

Someone I trust whom I can talk through this with who supports me unconditionally and nonjudgementally is:

Example:

A mentor from my support group.

What I intend to say as a part of my sincere apology is:

Example:

I've been feeling remorseful and sorry about jumping to conclusions and speaking inappropriately to you. I know you deserve to be treated with respect and kindness; therefore, I want to offer my most sincere apology about what happened.

The proactive solution I'll offer to help make it right is:

Example:

In an effort to make sure it doesn't happen again, I'd like to keep the channels of communication more open so we can clear up any mis-understandings before they get out of hand. I'm also going to talk this

through with a mentor and see if I can learn what needs improving in my thoughts and perceptions, so I can be even more empathetic and understanding of others.

When and how I plan to apologize and offer to make it right is:

Example:

This Saturday afternoon I'm taking my friend out to lunch to talk about this.

You can start with one specific incident you want to clear up and resolve and when you feel like you've got the hang of it you can take on a few more issues that you'd like to get off your chest and amend. Ultimately what we're looking for is complete freedom from any unresolved conflicts of the past. And of course, this is a method that we can all continue to apply in the future so we can properly deal with feelings of guilt and remorse, process them and let them go.

CONCLUSION

The ancient healing traditions within religious and spiritual teachings have emphasized the importance of atonement for millennia. Modern scientific discoveries are also showing that making amends can allow you to let go of negative thoughts and feelings, which in turn can help you feel better and reduce your risk of disease, depression and even addiction.

By following the method I've shared in this assignment, you can bring about deep, interpersonal healing. This is something you can take action on now and then revisit throughout your transformation journey. When you do, you'll be helping to heal and renew another person's well-being and your own.

147

transformation.com   transformation.com   transformation.com   **transformation.com**   transformation.com   transfor

13

What's So Funny?

Jerry Seinfeld is a healer. Jim Carrey, Jay Leno, Steve Martin… they are too. This is not just an opinion; it's a scientific fact.

The *New England Journal of Medicine*, in December 1976, first published a report documenting the remarkable story of a man who was healed from a painful and life-threatening disease by watching Marx Brothers movies and Candid Camera. (I'm not kidding. *This really happened*.)

The story of this man, Norman Cousins, inspired a book titled *Anatomy of an Illness*, published in 1979. Following his recovery, Cousins himself went on to lead a series of university research projects aimed at discovering the connection between laughter and health.

Cousins then went on to become a professor at UCLA Medical School and for the last 12 years of his life (he passed away at age 74, in 1990) he developed a research project called the "Rx Laughter Study" which explored how laughter affects stress hormones, the immune system and the disease process. This research is ongoing, now in its 27th year at the UCLA Norman

149

Cousins Center for Psychoneuroimmunology (the science of how states of mind affect the immune system). Among the findings of the research group at UCLA is that showing critically ill children funny videos, cartoons, TV shows and films greatly strengthens their immune systems. Researchers have also discovered that laughter helps the children heal faster and with less pain.

One of the professors involved in the research cited that laughter significantly lowers the "anticipated pain anxiety" which children experience when they know they're going to undergo an uncomfortable procedure. He says that laughter produces a remarkably relaxing effect on the autonomic nervous system, which controls such things as our heart rhythm, blood pressure, breathing and mental tension.

"The old saying 'laughter is the best medicine,' definitely appears to be true when it comes to protecting your heart health," explains Michael Miller, M.D., Director of the Center for Preventive Cardiology at the University of Maryland Medical Center. He and a team of researchers compared the humor responses of 300 people. Half of the participants had either suffered a heart attack or had undergone coronary bypass surgery. The other 150 were healthy, age-matched participants who did not have heart disease. All test subjects were evaluated to determine how they would respond to descriptions of certain scenarios. Would they see the amusement and laughter in them, or respond with anger and hostility?

At the end of the study all the information was collected and analyzed. It was discovered that people with heart disease were *much less likely* to recognize humor or be able to use it appropriately in awkward, even uncomfortable situations. Overall, they laughed less, even in funny scenarios and they displayed significantly more anger and hostility. This dovetails with additional UCLA data which shows a distinct correlation between misery, disease and premature death.

Dr. Miller observed, "The ability to laugh either naturally or as a learned behavior may have important implications in societies such as the U.S. where heart disease remains the number one killer." He continues, "We know that exercising, not smoking and eating foods low in saturated fat will reduce the risk of heart disease. Perhaps hearty laughter should be added to the list… exercise, eat right and laugh a few times a day."

Another expert, Dr. William Fry, Jr., has studied the therapeutic properties of humor for over 35 years. He explains that laughter ventilates the lungs and allows our muscles, nerves and heart to become warm and relaxed in very much the same way as exercise. Dr. Fry says laughter is like "internal jogging."

Humor is also good for the brain. When a person hears a joke the left side of the brain (analytical aspect) is activated. Then when a person 'gets' a joke and starts laughing, the right side (creative aspect) comes into play. Optimal mental and emotional well-being are associated with whole-brain activity (activation of both right and left hemispheres). A study at Johns Hopkins University Medical School even showed that humor during teaching and instruction led to significantly improved memory, learning and test scores.

Other studies suggest that laughter helps increase the flexibility and creativity of thought, which in turn, gives us greater ability to solve everyday problems while experiencing less frustration and anger. Make no mistake, the ability to laugh easily and frequently is a tremendous resource for overcoming difficulties, improving relationships, and building greater physical and emotional health. Scientific studies also show that being lighthearted contributes to the following benefits:

- Humor shifts perspective, allowing us to see situations in a much less threatening way. The lighter perspective often allows us to step back and see what's so funny about the things we do and how ridiculously serious we take ourselves sometimes.

- Laughter relaxes the whole body. While chuckling, our heart rates, breathing and blood flow go up temporarily and then, with the release of feel-good hormones like dopamine and endorphins, we feel tremendous

151

relief from physical tension and emotional stress for the next hour. This reduces anxiety and increases energy, allowing us to stay more focused, more present and more engaged with life.

- Laughter rejuvenates the body and mind. When we find something especially funny and break out in laughter, it lowers the body's levels of the aging hormones like cortisol (by as much as 39%) and adrenalin (by 70%). At the same time, the body's natural pain blockers and levels of growth hormone (the youth hormone) go up (87%).

- Laughter helps boost the immune system by increasing immunoglobulin A and gamma interferon, two of the body's frontline defense systems against viruses and bacterial infections.

- Laughter dissolves negative emotions such as anger and anxiety. It's next to impossible to complain and worry when you're enjoying something especially funny.

- Laughter helps connect people. Good humor becomes great in the presence of others who have similar intentions and experiences. In addition, there's a domino effect where joyfulness is passed from one person to another. It's easy to see how our good-spirited laughter can help others feel better too.

HEALTHY VS. UNHEALTHY HUMOR

There is a kind of 'humor' that does not produce healing laughter. And it all has to do with intention. When someone's actual motive is to ridicule, degrade, and divide with off-color jokes about religion, sexuality, race, or a person's misfortune, it's hurtful, not helpful. Humor that is cruel, cutting, condescending and aggressive produces the exact opposite effect of what we've been discussing in this chapter.

Laughing in inappropriate situations, for example: the loss of life, devastation from an earthquake or hurricane, or any tragic news is typically not a sign of mental and emotional well-being. What we're talking about here is good-spirited humor through relatively innocent observations, stories and jokes as well as, perhaps, getting a good chuckle out of our own foibles and sometimes silly habits. You'll always know truly positive humor because it brings people together; it lightens and unites hearts. Good laughter leaves no one out and produces optimism, energy and an upbeat mindset.

IT STARTS WITH A SMILE

Smiling is the beginning of laughter. And research shows that when people smile often, they're more open to seeing the lighter side of things and they experience much more positive moods. Ever try telling a funny story or joke to someone who clenches their jaw and scowls most all day? Right, it didn't work for me either.

Finding your authentic smile is a great first step. You see, you have a smile that is uniquely your own—one that's natural, comfortable, makes you feel good and brightens others whom you share it with. This is often called the 'Duchenne smile.' It's named after Guillaume Duchenne, a French physician who was conducting research on the physiology of facial expressions back in the 1800s. He discovered a difference between a warm-spirited smile and a fabricated one.

The real deal is apparent because it radiates from the eyes while the corners of the mouth turn up, rather than extend out to the sides. The facial muscles which bring about this expression are not voluntary (we can't make them move with our thinking); they're controlled by the autonomic nervous system which follows the lead of emotions. The forced or 'say cheese' smile is not your authentic one. In fact, that can often indicate something altogether different than joyfulness. When an animal exposes its teeth, which can kind of look like a smile, it's typically a threat or a warning display. In chimpanzees it can also be a reflection of fear.

153

Why did I bother explaining this? Well, a couple of researchers did an interesting study where they identified women in a 1960 yearbook who were beaming with authentic smiles. The researchers contacted the smilers at the ages of 27, 43 and 52 to conduct a standard life satisfaction and happiness assessment. By far and away, the women with Duchenne smiles were more likely to enjoy personal well-being and success compared to those whose pictures showed no smile, or a forced one. This speaks to another phenomenon called the 'facial feedback theory' which says that when we bring to mind something funny and we smile about it, our positive emotions and energy are significantly enhanced.

We were all smiling the bright way before we were even a year old. And it's likely we continued well into our childhood. Did you know that the average child smiles 400 times a day; the average adult, only 25? It's true. More often than not as we grow up and are conditioned by society, we somehow learn to curtail our sense of spontaneous joyfulness and penchant for laughter. But now we can see that reclaiming that aspect of ourselves would not only be fun, but it may very well help us renew our health and well-being too.

DEVELOPING YOUR LIGHTER SIDE

No two people express their comedic side the same way. Yes, you have a funny bone that's uniquely your own. And it's one of the most beautiful aspects of your God-given personality. To manifest more of it in our everyday lives requires that we move beyond the egoic self (prideful, defensive, judgmental) and take an objective look at the lighter side of ourselves. What we most always find is a reservoir of comedic material in our innocently embarrassing moments, the follies of our past efforts to improve or learn something new, our silly habits (everyone notices them anyway, we might as well get a laugh out of them) and even our mannerisms, including the way we talk and the way we laugh.

154

Another thing that really helps me is to keep reminders around my home and office which are there 24/7, reminding me to lighten up and have fun. I've got small movie posters of my all-time favorites such as Eddie Murphy's first Beverly Hills Cop; Jim Carrey in Pet Detective; Ben Stiller in Something About Mary and most anything featuring Steve Martin.

You may also want to consider putting together a video playlist of hilarious clips from YouTube and make time to watch five minutes of it every morning and evening. Check out theonion.com for hysterical videos to save in your favorites. Other videos which make me laugh most every time are the funny spoof commercials from past Saturday Night Live shows which you'll find at saturdaynightlive.com where you can watch them right on your computer.

I also keep photos around of me with my friends when we're laughing and having fun. And I very often work out in my home gym while I watch my TiVo'd collection of Seinfeld episodes. What about you? Does simply walking through the space where you spend your time make your smile, even laugh as you connect with a lighthearted memory? If not, maybe you'd do well to lighten it up in your own unique way. You don't have to go overboard of course, just adding a few photos to your home office space or bedroom can make a big difference.

Another important, common sense recommendation is to make sure you nurture friendships and connections with people who have a buoyant and bright sense of humor. Shared laughter is always twice as nice and the benefits always double. Make the time to see humorous movies, play games, and have fun with the healthy, lighthearted friends you enjoy the most.

What also helps me is holding the intention each morning of noticing the humor in the day ahead. Most every time, something will occur during the day that is completely unpredictable and totally funny. This awareness allows me to enjoy it and not miss it. So I always keep my mind and heart open, ready and willing to laugh at any given moment. What about you?

ACTION STEP

Based on the scientific evidence presented in this chapter, three specific health benefits of laughter which I am now holding the intention to personally enjoy are:

Example:

1) Reduced stress and more feelings of well-being.

2) Lowering my risk for heart disease.

3) Boosting my immune system so I can stay healthy and feel good.

Three moments when I completely lost myself in laughter with others, which I can vividly remember, and bring my awareness back to whenever I need a reason to smile are:

Example:

1) My friend and I cracking up on stage at the Denver Seminar where we laughed nonstop for about 20 minutes.

2) Our last family get-together where my brother and I started laughing at certain scenarios and couldn't stop.

3) The time I went with a group of friends to see Jerry Seinfeld perform his comedy routine in Las Vegas.

My five favorite funny movies of all time are:

Example:

1) Jim Carrey's 'Pet Detective.'

2) Steve Martin's 'LA Story.'

3) Eddie Murphy's 'Beverly Hills Cop.'

4) Christopher Guest's 'Waiting for Guffman.'

5) Peter Sellers' 'Being There.'

(If you don't own your favorite movies on DVD, consider purchasing them so you can watch them often!)

Three people I can connect with whenever I sense I'm starting to take myself too seriously are:

Example:

1) Friends

2) Family

3) Members of the transformation community.

Two times each day I can set aside five minutes to enjoy my pre-scribed 'laughter medicine' are:

Example:

Before my morning meditation and again in the evening.

CONCLUSION

Make no mistake, having fun is serious business, at least when it comes to the positive effects on your health. Your ability to rekindle your authentic joy and spontaneous smile is a wonderful sign that your transformation efforts are working. Sharing this lighter side of yourself with friends, family and fellow members of the community, who appreciate you and your unique style of humor, is a gift you should share generously. When you do, you'll literally be making the world a lighter place.

157

14

Addictive Habits

Chris Winters of Mesa, Arizona found transformation.com in the summer of 2008. He read about the program and decided he really wanted to participate. As he began to assess what it was going to take to get to the level of health and happiness that he was envisioning, he identified a problem. A big problem in fact. You see, for the last 10 years, Chris developed a very unhealthy habit of drinking alcohol, often. It had reached the point where he needed a drink of vodka just to get out of bed, and then he would continue drinking throughout the day.

This bad habit had evolved into an addiction. It became clear to Chris that for him to successfully transform, he was going to have to confront and deal with his situation. Inspired by a future vision of himself as lean and strong, confident and successful, and a good father and husband, Chris asked for help from fellow members of the transformation community who were in successful recovery from similar addictive habits. And it was there he first admitted to himself and others that he had become an alcoholic.

159

"I knew I wanted to get healthier. I knew I wanted to get better. But every time I would start it would only last a couple of weeks and I would revert back to drinking. I was so out of shape. My highest weight was 220 lbs. And the thing about alcoholism is that it's a very lonely existence. I had to turn things around, otherwise the end result was going to be very, very bad."

Chris continues, "I said if I can stay sober for 30 days, then I'm going to start the transformation program. The support I got online really changed my life. I remember the hardest part about that time was taking a revealing 'before' photo and sharing it with another person. That was tough because I knew I'd let myself go but I didn't want to face it. I got to the point where I was embarrassed to take a shower around my wife, or even dress around her. And then I had to ask her to take a before picture. It was even harder to look at it because you have to take a really hard look at yourself and say what has this person become. What have I become?"

Chris stayed in touch with his friends from the transformation community who encouraged him to also start attending local AA meetings. And before he knew it, he accomplished his first goal of being sober for 30 full days. Then he gave his all to the transformation program, completing all the action steps.

"Life now, being sober and being healthy, it's what life is supposed to be like. I've been sober a little over two years now. I have a completely different outlook and my body feels so much better. Everything about me is different. My life is not controlled by my addictions. The sky's the limit now."

You can see from Chris' before and after pictures that his condition has completely changed for the better. At age 41, he's as athletic and strong as he's ever been. He not only rebuilt his body in 18 weeks, but he was able to transcend his limiting addiction and renew his relationship with his beautiful wife and their three young children. One of the most empowering visions Chris would imagine throughout his transformation was being a hero to his kids. Now, his dream has become a reality.

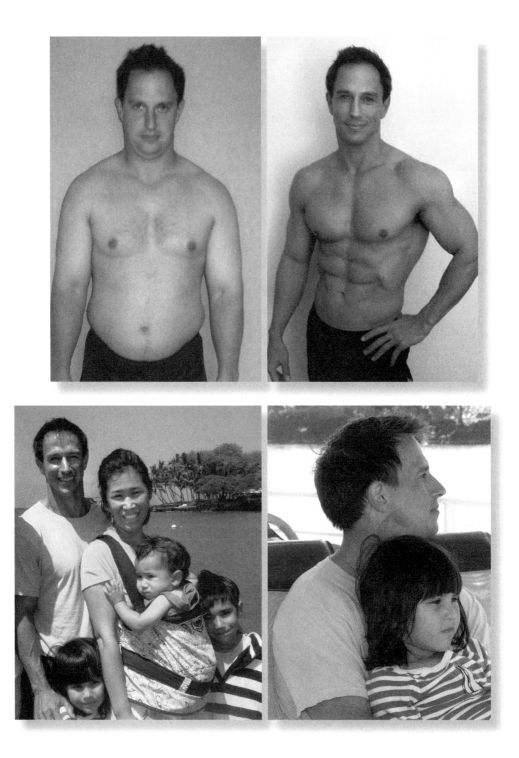

YOU CAN ONLY RISE AS HIGH AS YOUR LOWEST HABIT

As Chris discovered, breaking free from the chains of unhealthy behaviors can allow you to take a quantum leap forward in your life. But until you do, there's no end to the amount of time we can spend imprisoned, suffering and missing out on the full spectrum of what life has to offer.

Some people's unhealthy habit is occasionally eating one too many donuts. But most often, with people who choose transformation, it's something more than that. There are almost as many kinds of addictive habits as there are people. Yes, they include drug and alcohol problems. But more often than most people realize the substance of abuse can be something that seems so innocent... *food*. Numerous scientific studies have demonstrated that high-sugar and high-fat foods light up the same addictive centers in the brain as heroin. Fortunately, breaking addictions to food is typically less difficult than it is with such harsh drugs.

We can even get addicted to anger, complaining and self-pity because these emotional states release significant quantities of adrenalin into our systems. Adrenalin becomes a 'DOC' (drug of choice) for millions of people who don't feel comfortable dealing with their feelings and emotions. Unfortunately, numbing our feelings is not a solution to anything, it simply creates more problems in the long run. Our emotional states are rich with valuable information which helps us learn what we need to change in order to more closely align with our healthy self.

HABITS VS. ADDICTION

How do you know if you've got a bad habit or if it might be an addiction? You should be able to change the habit on your own. Whereas an addiction is a bad habit that you can't stop doing on your own. Addiction runs the spectrum from relatively superficial on one end to a deep psychic hook on the other. They present a physical, mental, emotional and even spiritual health challenge, and therefore require an integrated solution. From my 20 years of study and real-world experience, it's become increasingly clear that so much of the preventable ill health, depression and suffering that goes on in America today is caused by addiction.

What I've discovered over the years is that most people would have already stopped living an unhealthy lifestyle if they could. When we can't, we're not merely looking at how to make healthier choices; in fact, choice can have very little to do with it. When a person's bad habits become addictions, there is no longer much choice until they reach out for help.

The longer bad habits linger, the greater the likelihood is that they'll become a real problem. You see, for a while you can stop the drink, the puff, the binge, through the power of your individual will. Yet there's a point where we can truly say that the unhealthy habit becomes an addiction and your personal willpower isn't nearly enough to help you break free of it. Unfortunately, rarely do we realize when that transition happens. It can occur beneath a person's awareness. The longer the addiction goes untreated, the more deeply the hook is set.

Oftentimes people mistakenly believe that addiction is something that only happens to strung-out drug addicts and bums but that is very far from the truth. It's a condition that can affect doctors, lawyers, moms and Marines, as well as the world's greatest athletes. It can affect those young and old, black or white, heavy or thin, rich or poor; it doesn't discriminate. It's also important to understand that bad habits and addictions don't define a person. The unhealthy behavior is what someone does, not who someone is.

The more powerfully and rapidly a substance or behavior changes and alters a person's state—lifting their perceived energy up, calming the stress down, or mellowing the situation out—the more addictive it is. The hard, street drugs can bring a person to their knees, even force them to beg for help, in a matter of months. Many other unhealthy behaviors are more subtle and they can linger for years and years before a person really even recognizes the level of suffering the substance is causing them. This is especially the case with food addictions. Not only is it socially acceptable to eat unhealthy foods, it's highly encouraged by multi-billion dollar marketing and media campaigns which never end.

HOW DO YOU TRANSCEND YOUR UNHEALTHY HABITS?

First, we need to take an extremely honest and courageous look at ourselves, our patterns of action and where we might have reached sticking points before. The egoic aspect of our being, sometimes called the lower self or mind with a small 'm,' is often getting its needs met by the addiction so it can play some real tricks on us. This can be in the form of denial (Me, addicted? No way!); avoidance (I don't want to talk about it.); rationalization (I'm not really drinking/eating/smoking that much, and I can quit any time I want.); and projection (I think you're the one with the problem!). Although each of these arguments seem to make sense at the time, they're all methods the egoic self uses for defense.

Unfortunately, this lower nature, which we all have to some degree, is notorious for getting us into problems that it can't get us out of. It forms a sort of 'shell' that often needs to be 'cracked' in order for a higher energy, which greatly exceeds the strength of your individual will, to come in and help pull you out of the situation. And what weakens the hold of the egoic self? Truth. It can't stand honesty, its entire nature being one of falsehood. That's why every credible and effective method of addiction recovery includes humbling and sometimes painful honesty.

"Hi, I'm Joe and I'm an alcoholic." Introductions such as this will open over 10,000 support group meetings tonight across America. The reason they start this way is because this truthful confession allows a person's Higher Self to enter the room while it ushers the ego away. And you've already put this very same power into action in your transformation process; when we take a before photo, give it a good look with open eyes, and we share it with at least one other person, we're making a confession worth at least a thousand words. In an instant we move past denial and into awareness. And now we'll do a similar thing with our most unhealthy habit; we'll bring it out of the shadows of our unconsciousness and into the light of awareness, which is where the healing action is. Just this one single step changes so many things. When we're aware of our most unhealthy pattern of action, and we hold the intention to be freed from it and we ask for help, we're more than halfway there. And that's where I need you to be by the time you finish this chapter.

MY VERY PERSONAL EXPERIENCE

Unhealthy patterns of action are forms of adversity and one thing we can all know for sure is that adversity is simply a part of life; when we face its challenge, we often become better, wiser, more humble, happier people as a result. That has been the case for me throughout my life. Transforming negatives into positives has been my greatest source of personal growth and learning. And of all my accomplishments over the years, one that I'm most proud of is becoming a person who doesn't drink alcohol. Nowadays if I drink once a year, it's too much. But it wasn't always that way.

Golden, the town where I grew up, had about 15,000 residents at the time, and I think 8,000 of them worked at the Coors Brewery which is located right smack dab in the center of the city. If you were over the age of 18 and you didn't drink Coors beer... well... that's like being from Hershey, Pennsylvania and not eating chocolate. It was an inescapable part of the environment and a learned behavior passed down from one generation to the other.

I drank some in college (and tried quite a few different drugs) at the typical weekend frat parties but never let it interfere with my good grades and good workouts. And in my early 30s I ran with a group of friends (entrepreneurs and professional athletes) who all bought into the, 'work hard, play hard' motto. We'd work long hours each week and every other Friday night hit the local nightclubs and pretty much just get hammered. We never got in any real trouble and it didn't usually interfere with my work. It just seemed kind of funny in an immature way back then. But it had definitely become my most unhealthy habit and it held the potential to really screw up my life. At that age, with an exaggerated sense of self-confidence that was being fueled by ridiculous financial gains from my companies, as well as a mistaken sense of being bulletproof in my overbuilt muscular body, the thought of harm never really seriously crossed my mind. Looking back now, I'm extremely grateful that I made it through that era of my life okay.

When I reached my late 30s, going out with the guys and drinking wasn't the same. I'm not sure what happens with hangovers and age but it's brutal. I'm so glad I don't have to experience those anymore. Still, I kept doing it even though I knew it wasn't fun anymore.

It wasn't long after that my Father became suddenly ill with a rare form of lung disease. When he passed away at age 62 I wasn't prepared for the experience that followed. Those of you who've lost a parent can probably relate to a sense of confusion, the waves of emotion that would come out of nowhere, and the subtle feeling that a very important part of you is missing.

Now I recognize that void is actually an open wound to the heart and soul and it has to be properly healed with time, love and acceptance. But I didn't know this back then, and so without really even being consciously aware of it, I began going out and drinking two, three, then four nights a week. A few months went by like this and I remember waking up one day to a moment of clarity. I stood in front of the bathroom mirror, feeling a rush of guilt and shame and it was like my awareness was outside my body looking deeply into my own eyes and communicating to me that my Father would never want to see me like this. I made the decision, right then and there, to stop drinking

166

out of a respect for my Dad and myself. I've continued to hold that intention ever since that unforgettable turning point.

I humbly asked some friends for help and joined a support group of other people who'd made the same commitment in their lives. From there I reached out to get some additional help, from wise and loving experts, with the grieving and emotional healing process. For months I dedicated myself to this process wholeheartedly and not only worked through the pain from losing a loved one, but I also worked through the emotional bumps and bruises that I had experienced in the first half of my life.

Doing this work was incredibly transformative, and today I am the happiest and most fulfilled that I've ever been. My muscles aren't as big and beefy as they once were and I can't wash clothes on my abs anymore but I feel so good and my doctors show that my heart health is excellent. I think maybe in that healing process I kind of worked through whatever was making it seem necessary for me to build so much muscle. In the years since I made this important life change I've become both more understanding and compassionate.

Now I don't want to imply that my life is perfect; it's not. Since I broke free from that addictive habit I've had years where I didn't drink once, but a while back I also had a 12-month period in there where I tried drinking alcohol again three times. On each occasion it just made me sick. I felt that was good in a way because it helped me see that my body and brain had healed enough that they could no longer tolerate that toxin.

What I've discovered is that addictive habits sometimes really aren't that much of a problem until you hit some pretty significant adversity like divorce, bankruptcy, a health scare, loss of a loved one, etc. When we're down, they tend to sweep in and become an unhealthy and dominant force.

Of course, the best approach is to resolve the addictive habit before you hit adversity. In cases like mine, where that didn't happen, the next best thing we can do is recognize the pattern as soon as possible and reach out for help from a doctor or friend. You'll be surprised at how many nonjudgmental and sincere people are out here, ready and willing to help. The key is to drop the defense mechanisms, become humble, and just admit that you're having some trouble. To enjoy your full potential for health and happiness, please do the work necessary to break free from anything that stands in your way of that.

ACTION STEPS

After careful consideration, I've become aware that my most unhealthy habit I'd like to be free of is:

Example:

Smoking, drinking, overeating, apathy (being stuck on the couch), negativity, cynicism.

Knowing that if I were able to overcome this negative pattern on my own, I probably would have done it by now, I am asking for help from these three sources:

Example:

1) Your personal concept of a Higher Power or a universal intelligence greater than your own.

2) Counselor, doctor, addiction specialist.

3) A nonjudgmental friend, someone from a support group, and/or someone who has overcome the personal challenge I'm facing.

Three unhealthy feelings and emotional states that originate from my most unhealthy habit are:

Example:

1) When I overeat, I feel shame and guilt, then I mentally beat myself up for it over and over again.

2) The more times I 'mess up,' the more out of control I feel.

3) I end up feeling like I can't trust myself and I lose confidence.

168

Three ways these feelings interfere with my life are:

Examples:

1) When I don't feel good about myself I am less likely to show up at social events and sometimes don't even feel like going to the gym.

2) When I don't feel confident it effects my relationships and career.

3) Whenever I feel guilty I have less motivation to take care of myself because I think, "What's the use?"

Three conditions that trigger my lowest level habit are:

Example:

1) Bored or tired.

2) Stressed out or upset.

3) Lonely or disconnected.

Three people who will help support and keep me accountable as I work to overcome this personal challenge are:

Example:

1) Sponsor from 12-step recovery group.

2) Doctor, therapist, and/or a spiritual counselor.

3) An accountability partner from the transformation community.

Three good feelings I will enjoy when I break free from my most unhealthy habit are:

Example:

1) I will feel more confident and in control of my actions, behaviors, thoughts and mindset.

2) I will feel happier and my emotional states will be more steady and consistently positive.

3) I will feel like I can trust myself again and I'll be setting a really healthy example for my kids.

CONCLUSION

The work we'll do throughout the action steps in this book will help us heal and renew our emotional condition, set our mind in a positive, healthy direction, and strengthen our spiritual awareness and connection. All of these are essential components of regaining control of our thoughts, and behaviors. They're all essential steps in this holistic transformation process.

When you take away an unhealthy habit or addiction, you have to replace it with something better or you'll end up vulnerable to relapsing back to where you were before. You can also experience 'transference,' which is where we stop drinking but start smoking; we stop eating sugar only to find ourselves hooked on another form of junk food; we stop compulsive eating and take up compulsive gambling.

The reason this happens is because the addiction is really only a symptom of something deeper that's causing us discomfort, even pain, to begin with.

Throughout the 18 lessons in this program you'll be doing the kind of inner work which can heal at the core level of your being. When that happens, it often makes it no longer necessary to act out any addictive habits. And I can tell you from firsthand experience that this is both possible and quite remarkable.

15

Mind and Meditation

Meditation is an exercise for our 'inner health' that can allow us to live our lives in a place akin to the calm, clear depths of a tranquil, beautiful blue ocean. This is in contrast to the way so many millions of people experience life in today's modern world, merely skimming the surface, being shaken by the squalls, rattled by the chop and rocked by every wave. Most people lose sight of the fact that there's a much deeper reality to their existence.

The word meditation is derived from the Latin word *medi*, which means center. To meditate then is to connect with, and move into alignment with, the center of our being. It is going within and experiencing our true self or 'consciousness,' the Source which animates our life and is always there, quiet and wise.

Although our external self is very real in this dimension of life, our internal reality is equally important and perhaps even more so in the practice of true transformation. Turning inwards, becoming still, letting go of worrisome and stressful

171

thoughts, even for just 10 minutes a day, can help you begin living more deeply. Even while the external world changes faster and faster, and the surface waters swirl, when you know how to center yourself, you'll be able to feel confident, secure and strong most all the time.

MEDITATION AS MEDICINE

Although meditation has its roots in the ancient world, dating back 5,000 years or more, it's actually ideally suited for the busy and distracting world we live in today. In fact, it might be just the 'medicine' we need. And that's not just my opinion; the U.S. Department of Health and Human Services, through their research branch, The National Institutes of Health (NIH), began an extremely comprehensive study a few years ago to investigate the benefits of meditation.

So far, they've reviewed the findings of 813 separate scientific studies, some of which showed that test subjects who began a meditative practice and continued it for at least two weeks often experienced lower blood pressure, a healthier heart rate, strengthened immune systems and improved sleep (reduced insomnia). People also reported a reduction in muscle tension, backaches and pain, improved memory, and better cognitive performance. In longer term scientific studies, a significant reduction in relapse rates among those in recovery from addictive habits has also been documented. NIH plans to continue their research in this area.

The field of medicine called 'psychophysiology,' which is the study of how states of mind affect the body, is also interested in meditation. Their research shows that up to 75% of the people who go to a doctor's office or hospital each year are there because of stress-related conditions. And since meditation has been shown to reduce stress levels, it may hold the potential to help millions of people improve their well-being. It's safe, inexpensive, convenient and most anyone can learn how to do it.

Meditation is also used to improve mental health, specifically to help overcome depression and anxiety. Oftentimes those conditions are partially caused by mental stress, confusion and racing thoughts. Through meditation, what you're doing is actually taking a break from thinking which is somewhat akin to 'mental celibacy' where discipline of the mind is cultivated through consistent and intentional practice. When you do this, you are clearing and in a way cleansing the mind. It's a form of *mental hygiene*; keeping the mind sanitized is how it was described by the ancient Greeks. The word 'sanity' is a derivative of 'sanitized.' A cluttered, unkempt mind was the opposite of sanitized/sanity and was called *insanity*. Long before modern psychology, healers recommended meditation for most all mental health issues.

Those of you who are doing the complete transformation program, which includes regular exercise, healthy eating and all the action steps, are actually working on clearing the mind throughout this process with forgiveness, letting go of anger, confronting and working through addictive habits.

All these things, and meditation, work together to help you experience a very real and profound renewal of the mind. This essentially means you are doing the work to elevate your thoughts and motives beyond concerns of the egoic mind (externally focused, selfish interests) and moving into a realm of 'spiritual thinking' where your priority becomes serving the greater good, rather than just your individual wants.

A persistent myth about meditation is that it's exclusively for Eastern spiritual traditions. Although it is an important practice in Buddhism and Hinduism, it's also practiced in Christianity and Judaism. And it can be approached on a completely secular basis as well. So no, you don't have to chant the Lotus Sutra in Sanskrit or even hum 'Om' to meditate. (Not that there's anything wrong with that.) You really don't even have to have a religious conviction at all to benefit from meditative exercise. But perhaps what you'll experience from it could change your mind.

HOW TO MEDITATE

There are a variety of different techniques for meditation, but they're all essentially intended to bring about the same result. And that is to quiet the mind, slow down or even transcend our everyday thinking and gently access our innermost wisdom and life energy.

A quality meditative experience is one where you are completely present. That state is called 'mindfulness.' It is all about being aware of the moment you're in, while you shift to a state of non-resistance, peace and acceptance. When we're there, we become very open and receptive, which is important because it gives us the opportunity to listen to the subtle guidance from deep within. In effect, what we're doing is 'tuning in' rather than 'zoning out.' Rather than being drowsy or tired, proper meditation is done when we are very awake and alert.

The meditative state is a naturally altered sense of perception; one where you tend to lose track of time, feel a rich and vibrant inner happiness and are completely free of worries about the future and regrets over the past. This state of being exists only right here and right now. The thinking mind is constantly looking forward and back, and in effect, diffusing, even scattering our focus and energy across time. Through meditation, we can rise above that and experience the fullness of our true energy and intelligence.

Although the meditation I'm going to share here is practiced by sitting still, in a quiet room or a comfortable place in nature (park, by a river, on a beach, or even in your backyard), it's not the only way. We can enjoy meditation while walking, jogging, even lifting weights, that is, if our attention focuses inwardly through self-reflection. I sometimes workout alone so I can enjoy that experience. Remember, the second you start speaking to someone, you're immediately out of the meditative state because your attention shifts to the external.

Some people reach meditative states through activities such as gardening, painting or listening to music. One of my Grandmothers achieves this state through knitting and my Father's practice was fly-fishing. Whatever it naturally is for you can be greatly enriched through the kind of meditation I'm going to teach you now. I find that when I am consistent with this practice, I'm more likely to spontaneously experience transcendent moments and bright bursts of joyfulness during the ordinary course of a day.

GETTING STARTED

First, pick a quiet, comfortable place which feels good to you and where you won't be interrupted. Next, turn off any TVs, radios, your computer, cell phone, Blackberry, etc. If you're in a room, you can even dim the lights to minimize stimulation on the optical nerves which in turn activates the sensory mind.

Ideal conditions for deep meditation are often where we can experience 'sensory deprivation,' meaning that we won't be distracted by any sights, sounds, tastes, aromas, or touch. These kinds of conditions allow us to calm the mind much faster and more reliably. Also, it's best to meditate on an empty stomach, like in the morning before your first meal or in the evening a couple hours after dinner. You'll be able to reach an energetically lighter state of awareness when you're not weighed down by a full stomach.

The next step is to sit in a chair or on the floor keeping your spine and back straight (no slouched-over shoulders or arched lower back). Now, take a deep breath in, completely filling your lungs with oxygen. Breathe in through your nose, with your tongue gently pressing against the back of your top front teeth (to more fully open the airway passage) while keeping your lips closed and jaw relaxed. Your eyes can be closed or just slightly open, looking out at a beautiful view or a sacred object; a burning candle is often what I gently focus on while meditating, and it really helps me 'tune in.'

175

As you're breathing in, relax and soften your belly and let the chest rise up last, filling up from the belly first, like a vessel filling up with water. Your breathing is very important with this meditation technique. Exhale slowly while keeping your mouth gently closed. Breathe in for a count of five, hold for a count of two, then exhale for a count of three. Repeat this 10 times, filling your lungs more completely with each breath. With each exhale, become more relaxed, letting go of a bit more tension in the body and mind each time. Begin to see your attention as a soft golden light, about the size of an orange, and specifically bring that image over any parts of the body where you might feel pain such as the neck, back, shoulders or knees. With your awareness resting over the area, breathe in while you lighten the discomfort, and then as you exhale, let that tension dissolve and go out with the breath.

At this point, you can bring the light of your awareness and attention to a place right over your chest. Let each breath be natural and gentle, continuing to breathe in through the nose, letting the belly rise as you inhale and fall as you exhale. There's no need to try to force or overly control our breath or thoughts at all. Let it be effortless. Now, we'll gradually ease into contemplation (which is often called a 'concentrative meditation') where we consider a single theme such as gratitude, compassion, well-being, or joyfulness.

Utilizing compassion as an example, you would transition the light of your attention from over your chest to an image that represents loving compassion to you. It might be a spiritual symbol, or the first time you held your baby son or daughter. You could also see a family pet, or it could be an image of nature that invokes awe and heart-centered caringness.

Allow the light of your awareness to hold just one image. You may very well begin to enter a state of joyfulness and begin to smile. As you continue to hold the image you might notice random thoughts popping up. That's okay, it happens even after you've been practicing meditation for quite a while. We don't want to try to stop those thoughts; just observe them in slow motion as if they were clouds innocently passing through the sky. Bring your attention back to your image of compassion. Enjoy the stillness and continue to breathe deeply, gently.

When you reach the point where you're feeling the frequency of loving kindness and compassion, go ahead and let go of the image, completely clearing the mind and allowing yourself to be loving compassionate awareness. In this deeper state of meditation, we're not thinking or concentrating on anything and we're not holding an image in mind. There's no object or subject, just being completely in the moment, alert and one with the light of awareness, or consciousness itself. Again, if random thoughts arise, merely observe rather than identify with them, and let them float on by so they're not blocking your light which has expanded from the size of an orange to a light that has no limits. This is what meditation is all about. It's the center point or 'high point' of the transcendent experience. This state is often called pure consciousness because it's unobstructed by thoughts or limitations. It's like being in the full light of the sun with no clouds in the sky. This light is thought by many to be the source of healing, true health and well-being.

You may be able to enjoy that state of being for a moment, a few minutes, or you may just get a glimpse of it. And some days will be better than others, especially while you're first learning. It may take a few weeks to discipline the mind so you can slow and relax its thoughts and that's why it's called *practice*. No matter where you're starting from, you absolutely, positively have the capacity to achieve the true meditative state, and when you do, believe me, no one will have to talk you into making time for daily meditation; you'll be looking forward to it and you'll naturally make it a priority.

For me, this meditation is about 10-15 minutes from start to finish. When you're ready, you can end your meditation with a prayer or blessing, perhaps clarifying your intention to bring loving compassion to all your interactions in the day ahead. Then, you can begin to go ahead and slowly

177

open your eyes again, breathe naturally, and give yourself a few moments to reacclimate to the external world. From there you can move on with your day or you might feel like sitting quietly for a few more minutes while you keep all the electronic devices off so you can peacefully journal any insights that might be arising. You may receive some pretty clear intuitive messages throughout the next day as well. I keep a pen and a small notepad with me or nearby so I can write 'em down before I forget them. You might want to do the same thing.

Perhaps the next time you meditate you'll focus on gratitude, and another time, joyfulness or health. Utilize a single image during the concentrative part of the practice. As you become more proficient and comfortable with this form of meditation, you can direct it toward healing for someone who might be experiencing illness, loss or adversity. And you can also hold an image of your future, transformed body, allowing yourself to become one with the vibrant state of being which resonates within your new, healthy form.

ACTION STEP:

I am learning that proper planning ahead of time helps me overcome procrastination so I'm scheduling my meditation practice this week on these days and times:

Example:

Monday, Wednesday and Friday mornings before breakfast or in the evening before dinner.

A comfortable space where I can sit quietly and comfortably to meditate, without interruptions is:

Example:

Home office with the computers and phones off; a nearby park or natural setting; a local church or spiritual center between services.

178

Three themes and images I'm inspired to meditate upon are:

Example:

1) Compassion, with an image of my daughter the day she was born.

2) Joyfulness, with an image of how playful and happy my puppy was the first day I brought him home from the shelter.

3) Self discovery, who am I and what do I believe?

Three blessings, prayers and/or intentions that are important for me to offer after my time meditating are:

Example:

1) I will bring kindness and compassion to everyone I interact with in the day ahead.

2) I will allow the light of healing energy to flow through me today and uplift my friend who's recovering from cancer.

3) I will share this feeling of health and happiness with each person I interact with today by my way of being.

CONCLUSION

With regular meditation, you'll become more centered, less reactive, and you may very well begin to naturally experience deeper states of awareness during the course of everyday life. You'll be able to live more deeply, in the calm tranquility of your inner self rather than existing on the choppy and swirling surface. This shift is a profound transformation that can help you enjoy greater health and happiness most every day, in every way.

16

Heart of Gratitude

I will never forget the first time I sat down to talk shop with fitness icon Jack LaLanne. We met at a café which overlooked the beautiful blue ocean off the coast of Santa Barbara. It was a warm, sunny, summer-like day back in February 2001—the kind of day that convinces so many to move to California. We were joined by a reporter doing a story for *USA Today* about each of our perspectives on health and fitness.

Before the writer could even get his first question out, Jack looks at him and begins to explain, "You don't get old from calendar years," he said, "You get old from inactivity."

I smiled and nodded my head in agreement. The reporter quickly wrote down every word while he chuckled and asked, "How did you know that was going to be my first question?"

"It always is," quipped LaLanne before biting into a bright red apple. Our discussion was lively and fun. For two hours, we continued to chat about our views on exercise and how to stay energized and enthusiastic throughout life.

We agreed that virtually everyone is capable of transforming their health and well-being. Jack emphasized how taking on physically demanding fitness challenges has been a key to him staying motivated to train like an athlete throughout this life. The day he turned 70, Jack LaLanne swam a mile and a half, while shackled, as he towed 70 boats in Long Beach Harbor.

On workout intensity, Jack explained how, as people get older, they still need to give it all they've got. The writer for *USA Today* asked for clarification, "Don't doctors tell senior citizens not to push it too hard?" to which Jack barked, "What the hell do they know about exercise? Most of them know zero! You gotta push elderly people to muscle failure like everyone else. That's the only way the body responds."

Jack was 86 at the time, 50 years my senior, and still tearing up the gym every day. I remember thinking how I'd be happy to just be able to get out and walk on the beach when I reach that age.

As our time together was coming to an end the reporter asked us one more question, "What should people who want to live a healthy life do first thing in the morning?"

"Plan what you're going to do, or review the plan you've already made, and commit to it," I suggested.

Jack looked at me and smiled, gently shaking his head, letting me know that I've got a lot to learn, and shared one last bit of wisdom, "A healthy person always starts by counting their blessings."

THE SCIENCE OF GRATITUDE

What I didn't quite realize at the time, and obviously Jack LaLanne did, is that health isn't just a condition of the body, it starts within the mind and heart. What I've discovered since is that out of all the positive thoughts and emotions, none is more healing than gratitude. In fact, Martin Seligman, M.D., former President of the American Psychological Association, now founder and leader of the positive psychology movement, explains that his top recommendation for people who want to enjoy greater health and happiness is, "Count your blessings."

Throughout the ages, wisdom traditions, religions and philosophies have recognized gratitude as a key component of health, wholeness and well-being. Western science is a latecomer to the concept of thankfulness, but it's making up for lost time by conducting groundbreaking studies about gratitude.

Robert Emmons, Ph.D., is a professor at the University of California, Davis and author of the book *The Psychology of Gratitude*. Over the last decade, his research studies have made one thing remarkably clear: Simply being thankful can lead to a healthier, happier life. Dr. Emmons is involved in a large research project on gratitude and his discoveries include:

- Those who kept gratitude journals on a weekly basis exercised more often, felt better physically, and had a more positive mindset.
- Study participants who kept gratitude lists were found to be more likely to have made progress towards important personal goals (academic, interpersonal and health-based) over a two-month period.
- A daily gratitude intervention (taking time to focus on and write down things to be thankful for) with young adults produced higher levels of alertness, enthusiasm, determination, attentiveness and energy.
- Those who participate in a daily gratitude exercise have lower levels of depression and stress and are more likely to offer emotional support to others and help them make it through their difficulties.

In addition, scientific research showed that a group of adults with neuromuscular disease who participated in a 21-day gratitude program were found to have more positive moods, better sleep, a greater sense of feeling connected to others, enhanced energy and a more optimistic outlook on life.

A study published in the *Journal of School Psychology* showed that when children were instructed to count their blessings, they had a more positive

183

attitude towards school and their families. Another study, this one published in the *Journal of Personality and Social Psychology* showed that gratitude and spirituality are closely connected. In this report, grateful people were discovered to be more likely to feel a connection to others and something greater than themselves. This study concluded that gratitude does not require that you have a religious faith, but faith in a higher power enhances the ability to be grateful.

Dr. Michael McCullough, a professor at the University of Miami, has discovered that when people count their blessings, they are less envious and judgmental. Grateful people are also more generous and helpful to people in their social communities. One of his studies published in the *Journal of Psychological Inquiry* revealed that people with a strong disposition towards thankfulness have a greater capacity to be empathetic and relate to the perspectives of others.

The bottom line is, scientific research makes it clear that when we practice gratitude it helps us become more energetic, motivated, happier and altogether healthier.

HOW DOES GRATITUDE WORK?

That's the key question Doc Childre, Founder of the HeartMath Research Institute, has dedicated his life to understanding and teaching. The answer is in the heart he concludes.

The HeartMath research team has discovered that when a person is in a state of appreciation, their heart rhythm produces a smooth, symmetrical pattern of high vibrational waves. This, in turn, changes the way the brain, central nervous system and autonomic nervous system are functioning. Their studies show that frustration does just the opposite: it produces a chaotic heart rhythm, with jagged peaks and valleys which interferes with clear thinking and weakens the immune system.

184

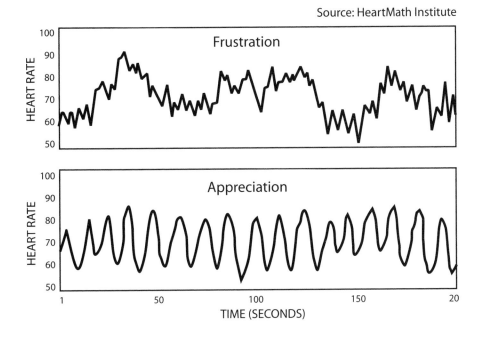

Source: HeartMath Institute

Researchers have also established that within the human heart there is a complex set of neurons (brain cells) that release neurotransmitters, such as dopamine, norepinephrine and serotonin, formerly believed to be produced only in the brain and nervous system. More neurons exist in the heart and solar plexus region—about 100 million—than in the entire spinal column and they appear to be heavily influenced by emotions. Gut feelings, butterflies, a knot in your stomach, these may all be the result of information being processed by the 'brain cells' in the solar plexus region (the area just below the heart and chest).

Intuition, inspiration and insight appear to actually resonate from the heart, in a literal sense. People who regularly find time to tune in and listen to their hearts say it speaks in the form of knowing (truth) rather than ordinary thinking. For me, relaxing and delving into a little meditation and detaching from all my thoughts for a few moments each day always helps me 'hear' my heart more clearly. Daniel Goleman, a Harvard-trained Ph.D. and *New York*

Times science writer, may have been the first to introduce 'emotional intelligence.' In his book by that name, Dr. Goleman cites numerous studies which show that emotional balance and self-awareness are essential to success in all aspects of life. He insists that emotional skills are at least as, if not more, valuable than intellectual ones.

Unfortunately, we learn nothing about this in the traditional educational system here in America. We learn how to perform tasks, how to solve math problems and memorize some basic information. We really don't learn anything about how to cultivate emotional intelligence and health, although both have more to do with happiness and success than perhaps anything else. Learning how to practice gratitude may actually be an essential element to a well-rounded education.

GRATITUDE IS A GOOD VIBRATION

The emotional energy of gratitude produces a high vibrational frequency. Negative feelings are a lower form of energy (termed 'lower' due to their slower rate of vibration). True health and happiness are high vibrational states. According to the wisdom traditions of numerous ancient cultures, the emotions of gratitude, joy, and love bring us into alignment with the energy of life or Divinity itself.

It's also taught that like attracts like and the level of a person's vibrancy at least partially manifests the conditions of their lives—the people they'll meet, the opportunities they'll have and how it will all work out. This means that when we align ourselves with the frequency of gratitude it will bring us into connection and communion with others who are resonating with positive emotions too. This is essentially the basis of the 'law of attraction' which many are aware of in the popular culture of today.

I mentioned this back in Chapter 4, yet I want to emphasize it again: HeartMath's research reports that the waves of energy generated by the heart are

5,000 times more powerful than brainwaves. This indicates when we're in a good place emotionally, our 'vibes' of electromagnetic energy produced by the heart are discernible and have an effect on everything and everyone around us. The opposite is also true. Again, if you've ever entered a room where people were having a dispute and felt it in the air, even though they were no longer around, you know about this firsthand. Ever walk into a cathedral after a spiritual ceremony and felt the loving presence? I sure have.

I always enjoy being around people who are living in gratitude because they radiate a kind of humble but powerful, positive energy. They're also much more present because when we're grateful it's comfortable and enjoyable to be right here, right now. When we're not living with gratitude, we're not fulfilled, not satisfied, and so we're constantly looking to the past and future to see if we can find what we're missing. Being in the moment is important because it's the only place where we have the power to change and transform our lives.

MY GRATITUDE PRACTICE

Jack LaLanne will be happy to know that for a number of years now, I've started each day by counting my blessings. I take about 10 minutes to quietly consider what I'm most thankful for. This ritual is a kind of casual meditation where I keep the computer and cell phone off and I sit down somewhere comfortable so I will not be interrupted for this brief amount of time. My favorite spot is on the front porch where I can sit in the morning sun and enjoy a cup of hot coffee or tea.

I start by taking a few deep breaths and I then bring all of my focus and attention to something that I'm very thankful for. For me, that tends to be the gift of life itself. When I quietly consider that I can breathe, walk, talk and laugh, it kind of blows me away. I end up with this overwhelming feeling of gratitude which I call 'awe.' I continue to contemplate this blessing for a while and remain focused exclusively on it. What happens most every time is that I feel an energy shift—I feel lighter, happier and inspired. Once I'm resonating with this healthy vibe I open my eyes and pick up my notepad and write down this blessing and a couple others I am very thankful for, and I bring each to my mind and heart.

I don't just think of a word and write it down. I let the feeling flow from my heart, down my arm and through my fingers, then the pen and onto the page. Every day I notice something new which helps me continually expand my awareness of the wide range of wonderful blessings I have to be truly thankful for. I always find myself smiling while doing this exercise and it helps set the tone for the rest of the day.

A second exercise that I've been practicing for many years is putting gratitude into action. After I count my blessings I write down two specific people who've made, or are making, a positive difference in my life. And before the day begins, I write them an appreciation message and send it by letter, card or email. I include precisely what it is that I'm acknowledging and I let them know the way it makes me feel.

I've written to schoolteachers that I haven't seen in years, friends from way back when, and I'm continually writing appreciation messages to family, co-workers, acquaintances and people from the community. Perhaps most important of all, for me at least, is to thank Divinity through both prayer and by living my life in a way that serves others and the greater good.

When you start your day this way, you'll immediately begin to experience more positive energy and within a matter of weeks, your neuronal circuitry, through which the energy of your thoughts and emotions flow, will begin to reconfigure. You'll start to become hardwired for gratitude and it will become a part of your mindset. For this to happen, your gratitude practice has to be consistent for several weeks. This shift leads to a kind of personality and energy change that will be quite discernible to those around you; they might even notice it before you do.

ACTION STEP

A specific time of day that I can consistently enjoy a little time to tune into gratitude is:

Example:

During my morning or evening meditation.

Three specific blessings which I'm very grateful for are:

Example:

1) It's a blessing to feel good, be alive and have the opportunity to improve myself.

2) I am very grateful for the support and encouragement of my friends and family.

3) I am grateful that many aspects of the transformation process are difficult because it gives me a chance to face my fears and become more confident.

Two people I will share a sincere gratitude message with today are:

Example:

1) My friend from the community who makes me feel like there are people out there who really do care.

2) My family member who's cheering me on and making me feel like a winner already.

This statement confirms and verifies that I put gratitude into action today by sending two letters, cards, emails or by thanking people in person or by telephone:

Example:

I sent my accountability partner a sincere email expressing my gratitude this morning and took a few moments to call a family member and share an overdue thank you.

189

CONCLUSION

Throughout the ages, gratitude has been a foundational element to spiritual practices and philosophies. Now, even modern science is coming to the conclusion that continually counting your blessings may be an antidote for negativity and stress. What's more, it's free, relatively simple and it's something everyone can do. When you begin putting the transformative power of gratitude to work in your life, it will immediately begin to make a significant difference in your health, happiness and overall experience of life.

17

Making a Difference

There is a remarkable connection between living a kinder, more generous life, and living a happier, healthier one. Over the last decade, this connection has begun to generate significant interest amongst scientists and doctors throughout the modern world. What they're discovering is very much what spiritual traditions have been teaching us all along: "It is more blessed to give than to receive." (Acts 20:35 [NIV]).

Could helping others be a path to self-improvement? Do we contribute more to our own health and healing when we turn our attention to helping someone else? According to recent scientific discoveries the answer is a resounding YES.

Dr. Frank Riessman, a distinguished psychologist and founding editor of the journal *Social Policy*, was the first to define the principles of 'helping therapy,' which is a form of healing that people experience when they make a difference for someone else. Dr. Riessman became aware of this phenomenon by observational studies of numerous self-help groups. A primary reason why they can work very well, he concluded, is because they teach that it is absolutely essential to be of service to others to help oneself. I often say that, "The best exercise we will ever do is reaching out and lifting others up." And according to another study, published in the *Journal of Health Psychology* (1999), we can pretty much take that saying literally.

In this report, a leading researcher in the science of healthy aging, Dr. Doug Oman, discovered that people who volunteer for two or more organizations have at least a 44% decreased chance of dying prematurely from disease conditions than non-volunteers. This same report showed that exercising four times a week produced a 30% reduction in death rates for the people in this long-term study. Remarkably, the results of this research revealed that not volunteering or regularly being of service to others poses a health risk as equally deleterious as smoking.

The Corporation for National & Community Service provides two million Americans of all ages and backgrounds with volunteer support opportunities. They operate AmeriCorps, Senior Corps and Learn and Serve America. They conducted a study using health and volunteer data from the U.S. Census Bureau and the Center for Disease Control and Prevention. Again, it was discovered that high volunteer activity produces lower rates of mortality and fewer incidences of heart disease.

At the Duke University Heart Center Patient Support Program, researchers found that former cardiac patients, who make regular visits to help support those recently hospitalized with heart disease conditions, enjoy a heightened sense of purpose, reduced levels of despair and depression, and a longer life.

In 2008, a leading British governmental think tank called 'Foresight' (headed by the government's Chief Scientific Professor John Beddington and comprising over 400 distinguished researchers) issued a major report titled 'Mental Capital and Well-being' in which a campaign for the improvement of overall mind and body health was described. A key finding for enhanced well-being and prevention of depression was, "Giving to neighbors and communities." These studies and others substantiate the contention that making a difference can increase our *quantity* of life, but what about *quality*? Well, there's a growing body of evidence to support that too. Solid, scientific studies show that when people approach life with benevolent attitudes and actions, centered on the good of others, it significantly contributes to the giver's happiness, health and fulfillment.

For example, in a study published in *Psychology Today*, researcher Allan Luks was the first to carefully describe what's been deemed 'helper's high.' Luks studied thousands of volunteers across the United States and found that people who helped other people consistently reported better well-being than their peers and many stated that the health improvements began right after they started to volunteer.

Not only that but helpers report a wonderful physical sensation associated with being of service to others. I call it 'sol voltage' as I've already mentioned. To me it feels like the pure energy of life itself. In the *Psychology Today* study, 50% of the people reported that they experienced *helper's high*; 43% felt stronger and more energetic; another significant percentage reported they felt calmer, less depressed, experienced fewer aches and pains, while still more reported that volunteering gave them greater feelings of self-worth.

In yet another scientific study, this one published in the journal *Psychosomatic Medicine* (2003) researchers specifically state, "*Giving* help was discovered to reduce anxiety and depression more than *receiving* help." I've certainly experienced this myself, as have many others I've talked with and done volunteer work next to.

Altruism is the virtue of doing good deeds without the need to receive anything in return. It's giving from the heart, with no strings attached. The fact that these scientific studies show that we do indeed receive when we give does not necessarily mean that our intentions become any less altruistic, in

193

the purest sense. And this is true so long as getting something in return is not expected, demanded or even needed. It's the non-attachment to outcomes which is key.

IT'S ABOUT SO MUCH MORE THAN MONEY

Sometimes benevolent generosity involves donating money and sometimes it doesn't. It appears that the most valuable thing we can contribute is our time, attention, and compassion. Dr. David Spiegel, a physician and Associate Chair of Psychiatry at Stanford University, conducted a research project which brought this to light. He randomly assigned women with advanced-metastatic breast cancer to routine care or routine care *plus* participation in a cancer patient support group which provided a safe place for the women to both give and receive loving care. Dr. Spiegel expected the support group would help enhance patients' energy and mood, but not survival. As it turned out, women in the support group, survived *twice as long* as the women without support. Participation in the group involved a considerable amount of giving to others primarily through attentive listening, understanding and empathy.

Even though I've been a proponent of, and an active participant in, supporting people directly and through charities in their time of need, I initially wondered if these remarkable statistics and scientific findings about the health and life-enhancing effects of being of service weren't influenced by some other factors. For example, at first glance, it might seem like a reasonable argument could be made that people who suffer from anxiety and depression would be less likely to volunteer than those who are feeling good and healthy; therefore, I thought these studies might merely reflect that people who are doing well are more likely to volunteer, as well as live longer, healthier, happier lives. However, the more I investigated and sought to fully understand the research, the more clear it became that getting involved as a helper or volunteer can create a turning point in one's mental and physical well-being. And while depression may be a barrier to volunteering in some cases, it's a motivating factor in others. You see, many people don't truly recognize the importance of making a difference until they personally suffer significant hardship through the loss of a loved one, divorce, bankruptcy, disease or addiction. In these kinds of incidences, reaching out for help often simultaneously opens a door to help support others who are going through the same or similar adversity.

Out of all the things I've learned over the years about health and well-being, I don't think I've discovered a better coping mechanism for personal suffering than getting actively involved as a volunteer, supporter, activist or advocate of a cause that you have genuine belief in.

BODY, MIND, HEART AND SOUL

Typically, Western science does not consider the mind and body related; therefore, standard medicine in the U.S. doesn't often recognize the connection between emotional and physical health. An exception is the field of psychosomatics (mind-body medicine). However, there's an overwhelming preponderance of evidence that the way someone feels absolutely affects the condition of their body. The most powerful form of preventative medicine one can practice may very well be cultivating positive emotional states of being. I'm not referring to hedonistic pleasures and gluttonous behaviors that feel good temporarily only to leave one feeling worse in the long run; but rather, approaching life with the intention of helping others and making the whole world a little bit better place, instead of just our individual corner of it.

What we're learning in this chapter is that we experience more positive emotions as a result of giving care and compassion to others. When we do that, negative emotions such as resentment, fear, envy, worry and hostility get crowded out. It seems that positive and negative emotions cannot coexist well within our hearts and minds. For example, I've never met a person who was feeling tremendous inner happiness at the same time they were plotting

195

revenge against someone whom they perceived had wronged them. Unfortunately, millions of Americans and others in modernized nations live in a perpetual state of negative emotion in part because they're in a chronic 'fight or flight' condition.

This is often in response to extreme and prolonged stress which causes the body to secrete adrenalin and hormones that prepare it for physical exertion (literally, to fight and defend oneself or flee to safety). This ability was obviously key to survival when our ancestors lived and hunted in dangerous conditions, exposed to numerous predators.

Today's forms of stress rarely, if ever, involve being chased by a tiger but our nervous systems don't completely recognize that. As a result, from dawn to dusk, people's hearts beat faster, their muscles stay tighter, their blood pressure is elevated and the sensation of fear is continually surging just beneath the surface. When people are in this condition, not only are they at a much higher risk of having a heart attack or stroke but their immune system is being constantly compromised, making them vulnerable to flus, viruses, infection and disease.

MAKING A CHANGE IS MAKING A DIFFERENCE

As you undoubtedly know by now, I see the deterioration of health and well-being amongst American adults and children to be one of the greatest travesties the nation has ever suffered from. Untold millions painfully perish before they live their full lifetime and answer their calling. To me, this is just unacceptable, and so I hold the intention of doing everything within my God-given ability to help put an end to painful living and premature death. In its place, we can bring health, happiness, energy and fulfillment. I've dedicated my life to this work.

Many people I meet resonate with this and want to be a part of it. That's good, because we need all the help we can get to make this great transformation from worst to first a reality in this lifetime. When people ask, "How can I help?" the answer is always, "First, change yourself." Start by becoming a healthier, happier, more compassionate, clear and energetic person. In doing so, you will make a difference in the lives of so many others, beginning within your own family. I've seen firsthand—there's no better way to help put an end to childhood obesity as well as depression in kids (which is escalating at an alarming rate) than when Mom and Dad do the work to become healthier and happier themselves. And it doesn't end at the family; your transformation will inspire people everywhere you go.

There's really nothing I can say or do (and I've tried it all) that is more activating than seeing someone you know make the kind of changes we're talking about in this book. It immediately flattens one of the biggest barriers that keeps people stuck, in that it allows them to truly see and believe that remarkable changes for the better are indeed possible. When they see what you've done, they really do begin to believe that, "Yes, I can do it too!" And that's a vitally important precondition to making the decision to change. By improving ourselves, we can each inspire others and make a difference in that way. In doing so, you may very well save someone's life, as well as your own.

This is the personification of what the great Hindu spiritual leader, Mahatma Gandhi wanted people to know when he admonished, "Be the change you want to see in the world." If you want the world to be a healthier place, be healthier. If you want to see a revival of kindness and compassion through our towns and communities, be kind, be compassionate. And if you want to make the world a better place, be a better person. It has to start with each of us. We make a difference by making a change and from there, as we continue to live it, we are indeed being of service to others.

This way of seeing things—this mindset—diametrically opposes the motives of both myself and those whom I helped early on in my career, back when I was in my 20s. Then, building ourselves up, going to extremes to build big, 'ripped' muscles had pretty obvious (obvious to me now) elements of narcissistic self-absorption. What's so different today is that my personal intentions and those of the communities I lead are the complete opposite. We recognize that cultivating a balance of physical health and emotional well-being directly benefits the greater good. And, neglecting ourselves—letting our physical health deteriorate while we chronically suffer from negative feelings—is actually a very selfish way to live.

When we settle for an unhealthy life, it adversely affects those around us and we even become a burden to the already strained national health-care system. In that respect, making time and making it a priority to take care of yourself is more selfless than selfish. And I can't tell you how many hundreds of times spouses and children of those who I help guide through the transformation process have both expressed appreciation and also surprise with how much that person's change has improved life for everyone in the family.

A TRANSFORMING COMMUNITY, MAKING A DIFFERENCE

Through the transformation community, people have the opportunity to connect with others who are open, ready and willing to both give and receive support. For those who've been through the 18-week initiation process, they can continue to grow by helping those just getting started on their journey. And no matter where you are on the path, you can give support and encouragement to those who are courageously confronting their fears and working through their adversities. Doing that is a form of service and compassion, which benefits, as the scientific studies show, the giver as well as the receiver.

Our transformation community is also actively involved in charities like the Make-A-Wish Foundation. Through our 'Running to Grant a Child's Wish' program we were able to make a donation of $211,000 at our 2009 event. Each participant collected pledges from others in the community and/or a few friends for each mile they ran in the Denver Marathon. It's such a wonderful experience for everyone who gets involved, with the high point being the moment we got to present that big check to the Make-A-Wish children and their families. I granted my first wish through the foundation back in 1994 and it was such an enriching experience that I've been involved with this group ever since.

Make-A-Wish helps make dreams come true for children between the ages of 2-17 who are facing life-threatening medical conditions. Through their work, they share an unconditional, loving and life-affirming message with the kids and families that says, "You're not alone." And, "There are people out here who care." Those energies, as we've learned, produce very real healing on every level.

Of all the things I've accomplished in my life that might seem significant, having been given the opportunity to grant over 550 wishes to date for Make-A-Wish children is the most meaningful to me. I also want others to experience this feeling too which is why my invitation to become a part of our ongoing Running to Grant a Child's Wish Program is always open.

You can learn more about how to get involved, in case you're interested, by visiting transformation.com. When you do, I guarantee you're going to be introduced to some of the most terrific, openhearted and healthy folks you'll ever meet, while you help grant wishes for kids who've simply suffered and sacrificed too much at such a young age. I'm sure, if you're anything like me, that's reason enough to get involved but I'll also remind you that your own well-being will improve, significantly, when you reach out and support Make-A-Wish, or any other charitable cause that your heart connects with.

BENEFITS, NOT BURDENS

A word of caution: Scientific studies also show that giving too much, to the point where it becomes a burden, can have a detrimental effect on a person's level of stress. For this reason, we all need to consider carefully appropriate and realistic ways for us to give. Someone who's working full time and also taking care of the kids might be taking on too much by agreeing to volunteer for 10 hours a week. Likewise, those who are carefully managing their finances to keep the bills paid and put food on the table should not feel like they have to donate any significant amount of money.

The scientific data suggests that there is not a linear relationship between the extent of giving or volunteering and health benefits. That means we don't get twice as much happiness from donating $50 compared to $25; we don't reduce our risk of heart disease significantly more by supporting 10 charities as opposed to a few. That being said, there is a threshold for experiencing the health benefits of altruistic action. According to studies that threshold is right around 100 hours a year or 8 hours a month. Much more than that does not seem to add benefits beyond the 100-hour baseline; however, I feel like we want to be careful not to take that too literally.

I'm convinced that the positive effects of helping and being of service not only depend on the time we put in but also our intention—the amount of heart and soul we give to the endeavor and the sense of meaning it creates. And let's not lose sight of the ultimate objective here. Yes, we might start by being actively involved in a single charity or worthy cause, but we should aim to eventually fully embody altruistic characteristics so they become a fundamental part of our everyday life—a way of being. It doesn't require any money or even any more time to generously, consistently and intentionally give kindness and compassion to others.

Offering a joyful smile while holding open the door for someone at the grocery store; giving words of encouragement to someone you see giving it their all at the gym; being a sincerely supportive person at home and at work. When you do any or all of these things from a generous heart with the intention of helping others, and with no expectation of something in return, you are being altruistic in a very authentic and powerful way.

ACTION STEP

Three specific changes I can make in my life that will make a meaningful difference in the lives of others are:

Example:

1) *Recovering and renewing my physical health will allow me to help other people who are overweight and feeling heavy.*

2) *Becoming an even more caring and compassionate person.*

3) *Breaking free from my addictive habit of (smoking, binge eating, apathy, alcohol and/or substance abuse).*

Two causes and/or charities which I genuinely believe in, and why, that I want to actively support are:

Example:

1) *The Susan G. Komen Foundation which is dedicated to raising awareness and finding a cure for breast cancer; it's especially important to me because my Grandmother died from this.*

2) *The Transformation of Health in America because I know what it's like to be trapped in a body that isn't healthy and doesn't feel good and I don't want others, especially my children, to have to go through this.*

Three altruistic characteristics that I can embody and reflect in my everyday life are:

Example:

1) *Compassion, which begins with how I treat myself.*

2) *Generosity, sharing what I can with those in need, with a loving intention and no expectation of getting anything in return.*

3) *Kindness, which I recognize has to include how I am with myself as well as others.*

CONCLUSION

Science and spirituality converge and agree that when being of service to others becomes a way of life, rather than a one-time event, you will enjoy a greater quantity *and* quality of life. People can no longer afford to believe, as individuals and a society, that making a difference is a discretionary option. The fact is, being of service in some way, throughout your life, is one of the most important and powerful things you will ever do for yourself and others. And that's a scientifically proven fact. So really, the only question now is: "To whom and how can I be of service today?"

18

Reflection and Awareness

Transformation is a life-changing process which begins inside, at the deepest level of awareness, perception, beliefs and thoughts, and radiates outward improving the health of your body, your relationships, and bettering your life circumstances.

In order to make that kind of change, we must work towards healing and renewal of ourselves physically, mentally, emotionally and spiritually.

By the time you've completed all the preceding assignments and action steps you will have experienced more growth and improvement than people typically go through in a decade or more. Now you have a profound opportunity to reflect upon and expand your awareness of just how far you've come. The more you actualize the lessons learned and insight gained, the deeper and more profound your transformation becomes. With that in mind, let's now take a look at your life in transformation.

You can read the following narrative in first person, as a series of affirmative intentions. So remember; when I say 'I' what I mean is YOU.

ASSIGNMENT #1: THE BASE AND SUMMIT

I am the kind of person who knows where I stand. I've taken an honest look at myself, inside and out. I'm not in denial about how I look on the outside, nor how I feel on the inside. I'm aware of my strengths as well as my need for improvement. I also have a vision—I know where I'm going. I utilize words and imagination to paint a picture of a future version of myself as physically healthy and energetic, emotionally healed and strong, mentally clear and focused, spiritually aware and connected. I remind myself where I started, and where I'm going, each day.

ASSIGNMENT #2: EXERCISE RX

More than ever before, I'm aware of the fact that for me to enjoy and sustain optimal health, I have got to keep moving. That's why I make time each week for consistent and vigorous exercise which dramatically improves the condition of both my body and mind. I see that so many of today's health problems, from obesity to depression to diabetes and heart disease, could be prevented if people everywhere would start exercising a few hours a week. I'm now leading by example and doing my part to help our nation transform from worst to first in health and well-being.

ASSIGNMENT #3: RIGHT NUTRITION

I recognize that when I eat right I feel better in every way. I'm also able to let go of unhealthy body weight while I improve my energy and fitness. I consciously choose healthy foods which give my body the essential nutrients it needs including: protein, healthy carbs, Omega-3 fatty acids, vitamins and minerals, phytonutrients as well as plenty of water. I eat smaller meals more frequently throughout the day to keep my body nourished and energized. This also helps me manage my appetite. I have a new appreciation for how important eating fruits and vegetables are, and I enjoy them often.

ASSIGNMENT #4: THE COMMUNITY CONNECTION

I've become aware that being a part of a supportive and encouraging community is a tremendous advantage. It allows me to accomplish things that I was never able to on my own. The people in my support group help me stay accountable so I follow through on the achievement of my goals; they listen and care when I share my successes and setbacks; and they allow me an opportunity to help them which I've discovered, always gives me renewed energy and inspiration.

ASSIGNMENT #5: LIFETIME INTENTIONS

I've given considerable thought to what my life is all about, what my purpose is and what I feel I'm meant to accomplish while I'm here. Doing this work has helped me become more clear in regards to how I want to live my life. With this insight, I've written a statement of my lifetime intentions. Now I have a beacon of light out in front of me which guides my everyday decisions about what to do with my time, energy and abilities. I share my lifetime intentions with the people I'm closest to so they can better understand what inspires the direction of my life.

ASSIGNMENT #6: HEALTHY SPACES MAKEOVER

I recognize that it's hard to do the right thing in the wrong environment, despite how much I really want to change for the better. And so I utilize my discipline to do everything I can to make sure I end up in the right place at the right time. I keep healthy foods in my kitchen, and very little, if any junk food. I make an effort to associate each day with people who have also made the decision to be the change and become healthier and brighter. I recognize that I don't always have control over all of my environments, but my most important ones, like my home and my mind, I keep clear of anything that doesn't support my health, my happiness and my transformation objectives.

ASSIGNMENT #7: PROGRESS NOT PERFECTION

I humbly and gratefully accept that I am not and will never be perfect; therefore, I focus on progress instead. I see where improvements are being made and I direct my attention to that, because I've learned that where my attention goes, energy flows. Each day I make an effort to see areas where I'm making specific, objectively verifiable progress. I also measure my success by what I have accomplished, not what I haven't. For me, success means completing the daily work which moves me closer to the achievement of my transformation intentions and goals.

ASSIGNMENT #8: THE BIG FORGIVE

I am becoming an unconditionally forgiving person. I recognize that resentment is a toxin to my mind and body. I'm now aware that letting go of grievances allows me to enjoy life more while also reducing my risk of heart disease, depression and even some forms of cancer. Any form of unforgiveness hurts me more than anyone else, and now, more than ever, I realize that's both unnecessary and unacceptable. Forgiving helps me heal and resolve the hurts and pain of my past which in turn, lightens and brightens my future. I know from firsthand experience that forgiveness isn't always easy, but it is always the right thing to do.

ASSIGNMENT #9: ACCEPTING RESPONSIBILITY

Instead of blaming others for the condition of my body and life, I've begun to accept that I'm responsible for who I am now and what I'll become in the future. I'm no longer giving all of my power away. By realizing that I am responsible for my thoughts and actions, I've discovered that I hold the power to change myself. I also now see that I'm merely responsible for doing the work to improve my health and well-being; I'm not in control of the results. So after I've done my part, I let the results be what they may.

ASSIGNMENT #10: THE POSITIVE MINDSET

My life on the outside is very much a reflection of my state of mind. Knowing this, I've developed the ability to nurture thoughts and perceptions that help me move closer to my intentions and goals. I see that the words I utilize to communicate with others and myself carry significant power. I now choose energizing, inspiring and positive words more often than ever before. I've also discovered that each time I follow through and take action toward the achievement of my objectives, it lifts and strengthens my mindset.

ASSIGNMENT #11: RELEASING CONCEALMENTS

I am increasingly more courageous and honest with myself and others. I've become aware that repressing uncomfortable feelings and trying to hide embarrassing mistakes from my past has a detrimental effect on my mental and emotional well-being. Therefore, I've begun to identify some of these things that I've been avoiding and instead of dodging them, I confront them head on. Then, I do the work to release them by confessing my concealments to a nonjudgmental, supportive person who is also doing their inner work. Every time I do this, it allows me to feel lighter, happier, more liberated, as well as more humble and confident.

ASSIGNMENT #12: MAKING IT RIGHT

I no longer let unresolved issues with family, friends and others weigh on my heart. Now I humbly and honestly admit when I'm wrong and I recognize more quickly when my behavior has hurt someone else. Whenever possible and appropriate, I contact the person who may have been offended by my actions and I offer a sincere apology. I also share my remorse and do what I can to make it right. I accept that not everyone is ready to forgive and that is beyond my control. All I can do is make the apology. I also make a point of forgiving myself in situations where I regret what I've done.

ASSIGNMENT #13: WHAT'S SO FUNNY?

Even though I recognize that transforming my health is serious business, I'm more lighthearted than ever. I'm aware that laughter really is good medicine, so I make time each day for a healthy dose. I'm cultivating my unique style of good-spirited humor and sharing it with others. I'm smiling more often and feeling a greater sense of joyfulness. I've also discovered that sometimes laughing at myself, the silly mistakes I make, and my occasional blunders, is a great way to let go of stress. It also helps me become more humble and authentic as well.

ASSIGNMENT #14: ADDICTIVE HABITS

I'm now the kind of person who courageously faces and works to rise above my unhealthy habits. I accept and I'm aware that any unhealthy behavior which I've tried to stop, but yet has continued to show up in my life in one form or another, is within the spectrum of addiction. Knowing I can't conquer these habits alone, I openly confront and confess them. I allow supportive, caring and nonjudgmental people to help me work through them. I am discovering that I can turn negative habits into positive lessons which help me live a healthier, happier life.

ASSIGNMENT #15: MIND AND MEDITATION

I'm becoming more and more aware that beneath my thoughts and thinking is a reservoir of wisdom. Through my meditation, I quietly observe my breathing and form a mental picture of something awe inspiring to me. For example, the rising sun, the ocean, a loved one smiling with joy. When I do this, my awareness expands and I feel as though this inner wisdom speaks to me in the form of feelings, intuition and insight. I'm learning to trust the still, quiet voice within, which gently, quietly, and wisely is always there to help guide me through my transformation journey and life.

ASSIGNMENT #16: HEART OF GRATITUDE

I'm the kind of person who is grateful for what I have, rather than being bitter about what I don't. I count my blessings to start every day and write them down in a journal. I'm aware that being grateful can help me live a longer, healthier and happier life. I also put gratitude into action by sharing a sincere and heartfelt 'thank you message' with at least two people each day who have made, or are making, a positive difference in my life. In doing so, I notice that I'm feeling more optimistic, confident and inspired. I appreciate now more than ever that counting my blessings is the right thing to do.

ASSIGNMENT #17: MAKING A DIFFERENCE

I'm making a difference in the lives of others by the way I'm living mine. I recognize that perhaps the most significant way I can help society become healthier, happier and more compassionate is to hold the intention and do the work to make those changes within myself. Being the change that I want to see in the world is a way that I can be of service to others every single day. Beyond that, I support worthy causes and/or charities which are near and dear to my heart. My life energy or sol voltage goes up when I unselfishly share what I have to give.

ASSIGNMENT #18: REFLECTION AND AWARENESS

I'm now the kind of person who sees and appreciates just how far I've come and how much I've improved. I understand that true transformation takes place within, at the level of my thoughts, perceptions, intentions and motives. From there it radiates outward making my body healthier and my life more beautiful and rewarding. I now see and feel the difference it's made to take a complete approach to change which includes not only exercises for my body, but for my mental, emotional and spiritual fitness as well. I'm proud of the fact that I've made great strides to fulfilling my highest potential in life.

ACTION STEP

The three most profound things I've learned about myself through this transformation process are:

Example:

1) I can take control of my life and change it for the better, on every level.

2) Even with my busy life, I do actually have time to take care of myself, my health and well-being.

3) I had the power to change all along and all I really needed was someone to point me in the right direction.

The three most difficult aspects of making the transformation were:

Example:

1) Taking the before photo and sharing it with another person.

2) Forgiving someone from my past who hurt me and releasing the resentment I've held onto for so many years.

3) Getting up the courage to admit I was wrong and apologize for something hurtful that I've done.

The three best things I've experienced as a result of the transformation work I've done are:

Example:

1) I've inspired my spouse and kids to become more active, eat healthier, and become more positive about themselves.

2) After so many years of struggling to feel good about myself, I can now say that I've forgiven myself, I love myself, and I look in the mirror each morning and am grateful and proud of who I am.

3) My doctor says that I've improved my health so much that I've reduced my risk of heart disease by 50%.

The three emotions that I'm most consistently feeling now are:

Example:

1) Inspiration.

2) Happiness.

3) Optimism.

Three empowering new beliefs I have about myself and my ability to transform are:

Example:

1) I believe and know through direct experience that I can accomplish important things that I set my mind to.

2) I am a healthy, positive, compassionate and caring person and always have been deep down inside.

3) There are many people out there that appreciate and care about me, and don't judge or look down on me for mistakes I've made in the past or my imperfections in the present.

Three specific, objectively verifiable improvements I've made in my physical condition are:

Example:

1) I've become 35 lbs lighter.

2) I can now run 10 miles whereas before I could only run 2.

3) I reduced my cholesterol 25% as measured by my doctor.

These photos are a reflection of some of the changes I've made in my body and life as a result of the work I've done to transform:

Example:

(Include both photos from the front and back, in a similar style to your 'before' pictures you took in Chapter #1.)

This essay of no more than 500 words tells the story of what my life was like before the transformation, my reasons for making the decision to make a change, what the journey was like and how my life feels today:

(In your own words, written from the heart, please share your story.)

CONCLUSION

Congratulations, you made it! You've met the challenge to confront your fears, overcome obstacles, heal your emotions and make some of the most difficult changes that a person can possibly make. I couldn't be more proud of you, the person you've become and the difference you're making in the lives of others and the world around you. You've gained significant knowledge, acquired new life-transformation skills, and by putting it all into practice, you've become more wise, more aware, and more alive than you may have ever been before. *Feel good; you've earned it!*

212

Conclusion

S o this is the end, right?

Not at all.

This is the beginning.

As I've shared throughout this book, the transformation is something that will help you profoundly change the direction of your life from now on. As you continue to apply what you've learned through the 18 chapters and action steps, your life will just keep getting better and better.

Myself and hundreds of other people have already incorporated the steps into our way of life. And you can do the same. You don't have to go back to the way you were before.

Just ask Shane Anderson, who three years ago accepted my challenge to transform his life. At age 38 he weighed 338 lbs, with virtually no hope and energy at all. In the first 18 weeks Shane became over 50 lbs lighter and began to feel optimistic about life for the first time in a long time. He continued for another 18 weeks and reduced his weight by another 40 lbs. And now, at age 41, he's still going strong. At a height of 6'2" Shane is now a solid 218-lb athlete who's completed three marathons and has more energy, confidence and strength than he's ever had in his whole life. He's inspired his three sons and daughters to transform their health now too.

Shane explains, "For me, it's not just about weight loss. It's about becoming lighter by letting go of the things that had been weighing on my heart for over a decade. This transformation for me has been one from dark to light, from selfish to giving, from apathy to action and indifference to caring."

He continues, "I'll never go back to the way I was before. My mind is different now, my heart is open, and my body craves exercise and good nutrition more than it ever craved pizza and beer. When you make the change within, it's yours to keep forever. I've literally got a brand new life now."

Shane's story is just one example of what many are discovering. When enough people make the change, we'll reach a tipping point, or critical mass, where a new awareness will flow throughout the mainstream consciousness and people everywhere will see and believe in their ability to change. They will be inspired to action. This is how the nation will be transformed from worst to first within our lifetime, quite possibly within 10 years.

Perhaps the most important key to making the personal and collective change and sustaining it comes down to one fundamental factor: we must all start living our lives *intentionally*, rather than *accidentally*. Not a single person I've ever met, in all the years that I've been helping people transform their bodies and lives, has ever once told me they became overweight, unhealthy, depressed or even addicted by design. It all happens when our mind and awareness are somewhere else. It's always accidental.

The solution is awakening to a new consciousness. One where you can see how each choice you make throughout every single day affects your health, happiness and well-being, for better or worse. With this expanded

214

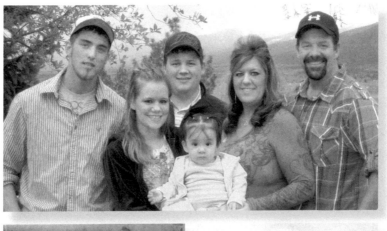

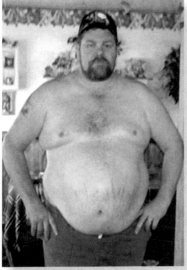

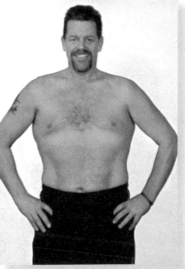

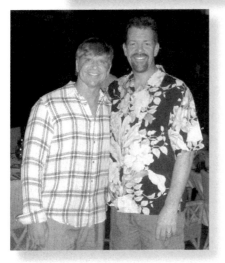

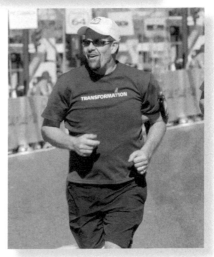

awareness, doing the right things to nurture your body, mind, heart and soul will become your natural way of living. That's the one thing that changes everything in your life.

By now you've learned, and even experienced, that extraordinary change for the better is within your grasp. In fact, you are capable of so much more than you knew before. And, as I said in the beginning, and now you likely know it too, all this time you've been closer than you might have ever imagined to being as healthy and happy as you've ever been. All you needed was someone to point you in the right direction.

As you've also discovered, you are not alone. There's an evolving, world-wide community of people who are waking up and discovering the power of transformation in their own lives, and how by making a profound personal change, they're making a difference in the lives of others. Our community grows in size and strength every day. People are connecting, supporting, encouraging, and caring about one another like never before. They're meeting in local get-togethers and building new, healthy friendships everywhere from Sydney to Dublin, to New York, Omaha, Denver, Detroit and Los Angeles too.

You've undoubtedly discovered by now that real change has to be an inside-out process. Anything that takes the opposite approach merely treats the symptoms. True transformation must include healing and renewal of your emotions, thoughts, mindset, intentions, motives, beliefs, perceptions and actions.

Now, you can see the link between science and spirituality and how both schools of thought agree that compassion, forgiveness, generosity, unconditional kindness, acceptance and understanding have as much or more to do with the condition of your life as anything else.

We can now see why just eating right and exercising is not enough. They are merely pieces of a puzzle which altogether, form the bigger picture of your new, healthy, happy, energetic and confident self. Putting it all together to transform

216

your whole person—physically, mentally, emotionally and spiritually—is the way to finally and completely discover what so many have been searching for all along. And it's not so much about acquiring something new from outside of you, but rather chipping away and letting go of anything which is in the way of your true inner self coming forward in its fullest expression.

No matter how far we've come, what you'll continue to discover is that there's always a next level of transformation, healing and improvement. Perhaps, continuing to move forward on that path is what life is all about.

Thank you, once again, for allowing me to share my message with you. And please, always remember, here and online at transformation.com, I'm with you each step of the way.

In closing, I have just one favor to ask. I'd like to ask you to promise me, and yourself, that you'll write to me when you're finished and tell me what's begun.

Scientific References

Chapter 1 – The Base and Summit

Matthews, Dr. Gail, "Study Backs up Strategies for Achieving Goals," Dominican University of California Press Release

Chapter 2 – Exercise Rx

American College of Sports Medicine Press Release, "Protect Against Colds with Exercise," October 6, 2009

Babyak, M., Blumenthal, J.A., Herman, S., Khatri, P., Doraiswamy, M., Moore, K., et al., "Exercise Treatment for Major Depression: Maintenance of Therapeutic Benefit at 10 Months," *Psychosomatic Medicine*, 2002, 62(5):633-638

Blumenthal, J.A., Williams, R.S., Needels, T.L., Wallace, A.G., "Psychological Changes Accompany Aerobic Exercise in Healthy Middle-Aged Adults," *Psychosomatic Medicine*, 1982, 44:529-536

California Department of Education, "Healthy Children Ready to Learn: A White Paper on Health, Nutrition, and Physical Education," State of Education Address, January 24, 2005

Cooper-Patrick, L. MD, MPH, Ford, D.E., MD, MPH, Mead, L.A., ScM, Chang, P.P., MD, Klag, M.J. MD, MPH, "Exercise and Depression in Midlife: A Prospective Study," *American Journal of Public Health*, 1997, 87(4):670-673

Eliassen A., Colditz G., Rosner B., et al. "Adult Weight Change and Risk of Postmenopausal Breast Cancer," *Journal of the American Medical Association*, 2006, 296:193-201

Holmes, M.D. et al., "Physical Activity and Survival After Breast Cancer Diagnosis," *Journal of the American Medical Association*, 2005, 293:2479-2486

Fiatarone, M.A., Marks, E.C., Ryan, N.D., Meredith, C. N., Lipsitz, L. A., Evans, W.J., "High-Intensity Strength Training in Nonagenarians: Effects on Skeletal Muscle," *Journal of the American Medical Association*, 1990, 263(22):3035-3042

Harvard School of Public Health, "The Impact of Weight on Cancer Risk," *The Nurses' Health Study Annual Newsletter*, 2003, 10:1, 4

Fielding, R.A., et al., "Activity Adherence and Physical Function in Older Adults with Functional Limitations," *Life Study Investigators, Medicine & Science in Sports & Exercise*, (November), 2007, 39(11):1997-2004

Folkins, C.H., Sime, W.E., "Physical Fitness Training and Mental Health," *American Psychologist*, 1981, 36:373-389

Holmes, M.D., Chen, W.Y., Feskanich, D., et al. "Physical Activity and Survival After Breast Cancer Diagnosis," *Journal of the American Medical Association*, 2005, 293(20):2479-2486

Landers, D.M., "The Influence of Exercise on Mental Health," *Research Digest*, 2(12)

Laukkanen, J.A., et al., "Intensity of Leisure-Time Physical Activity and Cancer Mortality in Men," *British Journal of Sports Medicine*, 2009

Lobstein, D.D. et al., "Depression as a Powerful Discriminator Between Physically Active and Sedentary Middle-Aged Men," *Journal of Psychosomatic Research*, 1983, 27:69-76

McNeil, J.K., et al., "The Effect of Exercise on Depressive Symptoms in the Moderately Depressed Elderly," *Psychology and Aging*, 1991, 6:487-488

Neale, T., "Exercise May Slow Telomere Shortening, Aging," *MedPage Today*, November 30, 2009

North, T.C., McCullaugh, P., Tran, Z.V., "Effect of Exercise on Depression," *Exercise and Sport Sciences Review*, 1990, 18:379-414

Ratey, J.R., *Spark: The Revolutionary New Science of Exercise and the Brain*, 2008, Little, Brown & Company

Trembblay, A., Simoneau, J.A., Bouchard, C., "Impact of Exercise Intensity on Body Fatness and Skeletal Muscle Metabolism," *Metabolism*, 1994, 43(7):814-818

US Census Bureau News, "Census Bureau Estimates Number of Adults, Older People and School-Age Children in States," CB04-36, March 10, 2004

US Department of Health and Human Services, Centers for Disease Control and Prevention, "Summary Health Statistics for U.S. Adults: National Health Interview Survey," *Vital and Health Statistics*, 2008, (10)242

US Department of Health and Human Services, Centers for Disease Control and Prevention, CDC's LEAN Works! – A Workplace Obesity Prevention Program

Willey, J.Z., Moon, Y.P., Paik, M.C., Boden-Albala, B., Sacco, R.L., Elkind, M.S.V., "Physical Activity and Risk of Ischemic Stroke in the Northern Manhattan Study," *Neurology*, 2009, 73:1774-1779

Chapter 3 – Right Nutrition

Al-Dujaili, E., et al., "Effects of Green Tea Consumption on Blood Pressure, Total Cholesterol, Body Weight and Fat in Healthy Volunteers," *Endocrine Abstracts*, 2009, 20:470

Anderson, H., Moore, S., "Dietary Proteins in the Regulation of Food Intake and Body Weight in Humans," *Journal of Nutrition*, 2003, 134:S974-S979

Antoine, J.M. et al., "Feeding Frequency and Nitrogen Balance in Weight-Reducing Obese Women," *Human Nutrition - Clinical Nutrition*, 1984, 38(1):31-38

Baer, D.J., et al., "Whey Protein Decreases Body Weight and Fat in Supplemented Overweight and Obese Adults," *Experimental Biology*, 2006: Advancing the Biomedical Frontier, San Francisco, CA, April 2, 2006

Baum, J.I., Layman, D.K., et al., "A Reduced Carbohydrate, Increased Protein Diet Stabilizes Glycemic Control and Minimizes Adipose Tissue Glucose Disposal in Rats," *Journal of Nutrition*, 2006, 136(7):1855-1861

Blackburn, G.L., et al., "Lifestyle Interventions for the Treatment of Class III Obesity: A Primary Target for Nutrition Medicine in the Obesity Epidemic," *American Journal of Clinical Nutrition*, 2010, 91(1):289S-292S

Bloomer, R.J., et al., "Alterations in Mood Following Acute Post-Exercise Feeding with Variance in Macronutrient Mix," *Medicine & Science in Sports & Exercise*, 2000:S58

Brinkworth, G.D., PhD., et al., "Long-Term Effects of a Very Low-Carbohydrate Diet and a Low-Fat Diet on Mood and Cognitive Function," *Archive of Internal Medicine*, 2009, 169(20):1873-1880

Crovetti, R. et al., "The Influence of Thermic Effect of Food on Satiety," *European Journal of Clinical Nutrition*, 1997, 52:482-488

Cunliffe, A., et al., "Post-Prandial Changes in Measures of Fatigue: Effect of a Mixed or Pure Carbohydrate or Pure Fat Meal," *European Journal of Clinical Nutrition*, 1997, 51(12):831-838

Deutz, R.C. et al., "Relationship Between Energy Deficits and Body Composition," *Medical & Science in Sports & Exercise*, 2000, 32(3):659-668

Dulloo, A.G., et al., "Efficacy of a Green Tea Extract Rich in Catechin Polyphenols and Caffeine in Increasing 24-h Energy Expenditure and Fat Oxidation in Humans," *American Journal of Clinical Nutrition*, 1999, 72(5):1232-1234

Duval, K. et al., "Physical Activity is a Confounding Factor of the Relation Between Eating Frequency and Body Composition," *American Journal of Clinical Nutrition*, 2008, 88(5):1200-1205

Farzaneh-Far, R., et al., "Association of Marine Omega-3 Fatty Acid Levels With Telomeric Aging in Patients with Coronary Heart Disease," *Journal of the American Medical Association*, 2010, 303(3):250-257

Fischer, K. et al., "Carbohydrate to Protein Ratio in Food and Cognitive Performance in the Morning," *Physiology & Behavior*, 2002, 75(3):411-423

Garrow, J.S. et al., "The Effect of Meal Frequency and Protein Concentration on the Composition of the Weight Lost by Obese Subjects," *British Journal of Nutrition*, 1981, 45(1):5-15

Gerdes, S.K., "U.S. Whey Ingredients and Weight Management," U.S. Dairy Export Council, 2004

Grimsgaard, S., et al., "Effects of Highly Purified Eicosapentaenoic Acid and Docosahexaenoic Acid on Hemodynamics in Humans," *American Journal of Clinical Nutrition*, 1998, 68:52-59

Hallahan, B., Hibbeln, J.R., Davis, J.M., Garland, M.R., "Omega-3 Fatty Acid Supplementation in Patients with Recurrent Self-Harm," *British Journal of Psychiatry*, 2007, 190:118-122

Harris, W.S., et al., "Omega-6 Fatty Acids and Risk for Cardiovascular Disease: A Science Advisory From the AHA Nutrition Subcommittee of the Council on Nutrition, Physical Activity, and Metabolism" *Circulation*, 2009; 119(6): 902

Harvard School of Public Health, "Vegetables and Fruits: Get Plenty Every Day," *The Nutrition Source*

Harvard School of Public Health, "Vitamin D and Health," *The Nutr. Source*

Hibbeln, J.R., et al., "Omega-3 Status and Cerebrospinal Fluid Corticotrophin Releasing Hormone in Perpetrators of Domestic Violence," *Biological Psychiatry*, 2004, 56:895-897

Hipkiss, A.R., "Glycation, Aging and Carnosine: Are Carnivorous Diets Beneficial?" *Mechanisms of Aging and Development*, 2005, 126(10):1034-1039

Jenkins, D.J. et al., "Nibbling Versus Gorging: Metabolic Advantages of Increased Meal Frequency," *New England Journal of Med.*, 1989, 321(14):929-934

Johnston, C., "Functional Foods as Modifiers of Cardiovascular Disease," *American Journal of Lifestyle Medicine*, 2009, 3(1 suppl):39S-43S

"Fatty Acids—Good for the Brain, Good for Alzheimer Disease," *Journal of Clinical Investigation*, 2005, 115(10):2585

Kelley, D.S., et al., "DHA Supplementation Decreases Serum C-Reactive Protein and Other Markers of Inflammation in Hypertriglyceridemic Men," *Journal of Nutrition*, 2009, 139(3):495-501

Ka-Hung, N.G., Meyer, B.J., Reece, L., Sinn, N., "Dietary Polyunsaturated Fatty Acid Intakes in Children with ADHD Symptoms," *British Journal of Nutrition*, 2009, 102:1635-1641

Kleiner, S.M., "Water: An Essential But Overlooked Nutrient," *Journal of the American Diabetic Association*, 1999, 99(2):200-206

Krieger, J.W., Sitren, H.S., et al., "Effects of Variation in Protein and Carbohydrate Intake on Body Mass and Composition During Energy Restriction: A Meta-Regression," *American Journal of Clinical Nutrition*, 2006, 83:260-274

Kris-Etherton, P.M., et al., "Fish Consumption, Fish Oil, Omega-3 Fatty Acids, and Cardiovascular Disease," Circulation, 2002, 2747-2751

Layman, D.K., Evans, E.M., Erickson, D., et al., "A Moderate-Protein Diet Produces Sustained Weight Loss and Long-Term Changes in Body Composition and Blood Lipids in Obese Adults," *Journal of Nutrition*, 2009, 139(3):514-521

223

Layman, D.K., Boileau, R.A., et al., "A Reduced Ratio of Dietary Carbohydrate to Protein Improves Body Composition and Blood Lipid Profiles during Weight Loss in Adult Women," *Journal of Nutrition*, 2003, 133:411-417

Layman, D.K., Baum., J.I., "Dietary Protein Impact on Glycemic Control during Weight Loss," *Journal of Nutrition*, 2004, 134(4):968S-973S

Layman, D.K., Shiue, H., Sather, C., Erickson, D.J., Baum, J., "Increased Dietary Protein Modifies Glucose and Insulin Homeostasis in Adult Women during Weight Loss," *Journal of Nutrition*, February 1, 2003, 133(2):405-410

Layman, D.K., Ph.D., "Protein Quantity and Quality at Levels above the RDA Improves Adult Weight Loss," *Journal of the American College of Nutrition*, 2004, 23(6):631S-636S

Lemieux, S., et al., "Seven-Year Changes in Body Fat and Visceral Adipose Tissue in Women. Association with Indexes of Plasma Glucose-Insulin Homeostasis," *Diabetes Care*, September 1996, 19(9):983-991

Liu, R.H., "Potential Synergy of Phytochemicals in Cancer Prevention: Mechanism of Action," *Journal of Nutrition*, 2004, 134(12 Suppl):3479S-3485S

Looker, A.C., et al., "Serum 25-hydroxyvitamin D Status of the US Population: 1988-1994 Compared with 2000-2004," *American Journal of Clinical Nutrition*," 2008, 88:1519-1527

Markus, C.R. et al., "Whey Protein Rich in Alpha-Lactalbumin Increases the Ratio of Plasma Tryptophan to the Sum of the Other Large Neutral Amino Acids and Improves Cognitive Performance in Stress-Vulnerable Subjects," *American Journal of Clinical Nutrition*, 2002, 75:1051-1056

Mayo Foundation for Medical Education and Research, "Omega-3 Fatty Acids, Fish Oil, Alpha-Linolenic Acid," 2010

Merchant, A.T., Anand, S.S., et al., "Protein Intake Is Inversely Associated with Abdominal Obesity in a Multi-Ethnic Population," *Journal of Nutrition*, 2005, 135(5):1196-1201

Meyer, K.A., et al., "Carbohydrates, Dietary Fiber, and Incident Type 2 Diabetes in Older Women," *American Journal of Clinical Nutrition*, 2000; 71(4): 921

Mozaffarian, D., "Fish and n-3 Fatty Acids for the Prevention of Fatal Coronary Heart Disease and Sudden Cardiac Death," *American Journal of Clinical Nutrition*, 2008, 87(6):1991S-1996S

Noakes, M., Keogh, J.B., et al., "Effect of an Energy-Restricted, High-Protein, Low-Fat Diet Relative to a Conventional High-Carbohydrate, Low-Fat Diet on Weight Loss, Body Composition, Nutritional Status," *American Journal of Clinical Nutrition*, 2005, 81:1298-1306

Paddon-Jones, D., Westman, E., et al., "Protein, Weight Management, and Satiety," *American Journal of Clinical Nutrition*, 2008, 87(suppl):1558S-1561S

Park, S.K., et al. "Fruit, Vegetable, and Fish Consumption and Heart Rate Variability: The Veterans Administration Normative Aging Study," *American Journal of Clinical Nutrition*, 2009, 89(3):778-786

Phinney, K.W., "Development of a Standard Reference Material for Vitamin D in Serum," *American Journal of Clinical Nutrition*, 2008, 88(suppl):511S

Poppitt, S.D., et al., "Effects of Moderate-Dose Omega-3 Fish Oil on Cardiovascular Factors and Mood After Ischemic Stroke: A Randomized, Controlled Trial," *Stroke*, 2009, 40(11):3485-3492

Radin D.I., Hayssen G., Walsh J., "Effects of Intentionally Enhanced Chocolate on Mood," *Explore: The Journal of Science and Healing. 2007*, 3:485-492

Rao, A.V., Rao, L.G., "Carotenoids and Human Health," *Pharmacological Research*, 2007, 55(3):207-216

Simopoulos, A.P., "n-3 Fatty Acids and Human Health: Defining Strategies for Public Policy," *Lipids*, 2001, 36:S83-S89

Speechly, D.P. et al., "Acute Appetite Reduction Associated with an Increased Frequency of Eating in Obese Males," *International Journal of Obesity-related Metabolic Disorder*, 1999, 23(11):1151-1159

Stevens, L.J., et al., "Essential Fatty Acid Metabolism in Boys with ADHD," *American Journal of Clinical Nutrition*, 1995, 62:761-768

Tanskanen, A., M.D., et al. "Fish Consumption and Depressive Symptoms in the General Population in Finland," *Psychiatric Services*, 2001, 52:529-531

225

Thielecke, F., et al., "Epigallocatechin-3-gallate and Post-Prandial Fat Oxidation in Overweight/Obese Male Volunteers: A Pilot Study," *European Journal of Clinical Nutrition*, 2010

Torpy, J.M., Lynm, C., Glass, R.M., "Eating Fish: Health Benefits and Risks," *Journal of the American Medical Association*, 2006, 296(15):1926

US Department of Agriculture, Economic Research Service," Patterns of Caloric Intake and Body Mass Index Among U.S. Adults," 2002

US Department of Health and Human Services, Centers for Disease Control and Prevention, "25-Hydroxyvitamin D Analysis," *The National Health and Nutrition Examination Survey*, 1988-1994, 2000-2006

US Food and Drug Administration, "Mercury in Fish: Cause for Concern?" *FDA Consumer*, 1994, 28 (September)

US Food and Drug Administration, Center for Food Safety and Applied Nutrition, Office of Seafood, "Mercury Levels in Seafood Species," 2001

Van Loon, L.J.C. et al., "Ingestion of Protein Hydrolysate and Amino Acid-Carbohydrate Mixtures Increases Post-Exercise Plasma Insulin Responses in Men," *Journal of Nutrition*, 2000, 130:2508-2513.

Venables, M.C., et al. "Green Tea Extract Ingestion, Fat Oxidation, and Glucose Tolerance in Healthy Humans," *American Journal of Clinical Nutrition*, 2008, 87(3):778-784

Verboeket-van de Venne, W.P. et al., "Influence of the Feeding Frequency on Nutrient Utilization in Man: Consequences for Energy Metabolism," *European Journal of Clinical Nutrition*, 1991, 45(3):161-169

Weigle, D.S., Breen, P.A., et al., "A High-Protein Diet Induces Sustained Reductions in Appetite, ad libitum Caloric Intake, and Body Weight," *American Journal of Clinical Nutrition*, 2005, 82:41-48

Chapter 4 – The Community Connection

Kornblum, J., "Study: 25% of Americans Have No One to Confide In," *USA Today*, June 22, 2006

Maslow, A.H., "A Theory of Human Motivation," *Psychological Review*, 50: 370-396

McCraty, R. Ph.D., *The Energetic Heart: Bioelectromagnetic Interactions Within and Between People*, HeartMath Institute

Rich, S., "U.S. Ranks 6th in Quality of Life: Japan is 1st," *The Washington Post*, May 18, 1993

Ruden, R. M.D., Ph.D., *The Craving Brain: The BioBalance Approach to Controlling Addictions*, 1997, HarperCollins.

Sacks FM, Bray GA, Carey VJ, et al., "Comparison of Weight-Loss Diets with Different Compositions of Fat, Protein, and Carbohydrates," *New England Journal of Medicine*, 2009, 360:859-873.

Spiegel, D. et al, "Effects of Supportive-Expressive Group Therapy on Survival of Patients with Metastatic Breast Cancer," *CANCER*, July 23, 2007

Chapter 5 – Lifetime Intentions

Haggard, P., Libet, B., "Conscious Intention and Brain Activity," *Journal of Consciousness Studies*, 2001, 18:47-64

King, L.A., "The Health Benefits of Writing About Life Goals," *Personality and Social Psychology Bulletin*, 2001, 27:798-807

McTaggart, L., *The Intention Experiment: Using Your Thoughts to Change Your Life and the World*, 2007, Free Press.

Chapter 6 – Healthy Spaces Makeover

Haggard, P., et al., "Conscious Intention and Brain Activity," *Journal of Consciousness Studies*, 2001, 8:47-64

Lau, H.C., et al., "Attention to Intention," *Science*, 2004, 303(5661):1208-1210

Radin, D., *The Conscious Universe*, 2009, HarperOne

Radin, D. I. (2006). *Entangled Minds: Extrasensory experiences in a Quantum Reality*, New York: Simon & Schuster (Paraview Pocket Books)

Rein, G., PhD, et al., "The Physiological and Psychological Effects of Compassion and Anger," *Journal of Advancement in Medicine*, 1995, 8(2):87-105

Wicke, R. W., Ph.D., "Effects of Music and Sound on Human Health," *Herbalist Review*, 2002, #1

Chapter 8 – The Big Forgive

Kendall, R.T., *Total Forgiveness*, 2002, Lake Mary, FL: Charisma House

Kitchen, A., "Forgiveness: A Key to Better Health," *Vibrant Life*, 2001

Luskin, F., *Forgiveness for Good*, 2002, New York: HarperCollins

Moller, J., Theorell, T., et al., "Work Related Stressful Life Events and the Risk of Myocardial Infarction. Case-Control and Case-Crossover Analyses Within the Stockholm Heart Epidemiology Programme (SHEEP)," *Journal of Epidemiology and Community Health*, 2009, 59(1), 23-30

Stanford University, Stanford Center for Research in Disease Prevention, "The Stanford Forgiveness Project"

Vanoyen Witvliet, C. (2001), "Forgiveness and Health: Review and Reflection on a Matter of Faith, Feelings, and Physiology," *Journal of Psychology and Theology*, Vol. 29

Chapter 10 – The Positive Mindset

Bem, D.J., Honorton, C., "Does Psi Exist? Replicable Evidence for an Anomalous Process of Information Transfer," *Psychological Bulletin*, 115:4-18

Bender, H., "Hans Berger and an Energetic Theory of Telepathy," *Zeitschrift fur Parapsychologie und Grenzgebiete der Psychologie*, 1963, 6(2/3):182-191

Colwell, J., et al., "The Ability to Detect Unseen Staring: A Literature Review and Empirical Tests," *British Journal of Psychology*, 2000, 91:71-85

Chapter 11 - Releasing Concealments

Cohen, S., et al., "Psychological Stress and Susceptibility to the Common Cold," *New England Journal of Medicine*, 1991, 325:606-612

Epstein, E.M., et al., "Getting to the Heart of the Matter: Written disclosure, Gener, and Heart Rate," *Psychosomatic Medicine*, 2005, 67:413-419

Hafen, B., et al., *The Health Effects of Attitudes, Emotions, and Relationships*, 1992, Provo, Utah: EMS Associates

Magai, C., et al., "Sharing the Good, Sharing the Bad: The Benefits of Emotional Self-Disclosure," *Journal of Aging and Health*, 2009, 21:286-313

Paterniti, S., et al., "Sustained Anxiety in a Four-Year Progression of Carotid Atherosclerosis," *Arteriosclerosis, Thrombosis and Vascular Biology,*" 2001, 36:21-136

Pennebaker, J.W., "Writing About Emotional Experiences as a Therapeutic Process," *Psychological Science,* 1997, 8(3):162-166

Sternberg, E.M., et al., "The Mind-Body Interaction in Disease," *Scientific American* special issue, 1997, 8-15

Selye, H., *The Stress of Life,* 1956, McGraw Hill

Chapter 12 – Making it Right

Cohen, G.E., et al., "Psychological Stress and Antibody Response to Immunization: A Critical Review of the Human Literature," *Psychosomatic Medicine,* 2001, 63:7-18

Lacey, J., Lacey, B., "Some Autonomic-Central Nervous System Interrelationships," found in P. Black, *Physiological Correlates of Emotions,* 1970, New York: Academic Press, 205-275

Radzik, L., *Making Amends: Atonement in Morality,* 2009, Oxford University Press

Dickerson, S.S., Kemeny, M.E., et al., "Immunological Effects of Induced Shame and Guilt," *Psychosomatic Medicine, 2004,* 66:124-131.

Chapter 13 – What's So Funny?

Berk, L., et al., "Neuroendocrine and Stress Hormone Changes During Mirthful Laughter," *The American Journal of the Medical Sciences,* 1989, 298:390

Cousins, W., "Anatomy of an Illness (As Perceived by the Patient), *New England Journal of Medicine,* 1976, 295(26):1458-1463.

Fry, W.F., *Advances in Humor and Psychotherapy,* 1993, Prof. Resource Exchange

Gibson, L., *Laughter, the Universal Language,* 1990, New York: Pegasus Expressions

Harker, L., Keltner, D., "Expressions of Positive Emotion in Women's College Yearbook Pictures and Their Relationship to Personality and Life Outcomes," *Journal of Personality and Social Psychology,* 2001, 80:112-124

Murray, M. W. (2009), "Laughter is the 'Best Medicine' for Your Heart," University of Maryland Medical Center

Chapter 15 – Mind and Meditation

National Institutes of Health, "Meditation: An Introduction," NCCAM Pub. No. D308

WebMD, Health and Balance Center, "Effects of Stress on your Body," March 8, 2010

Chapter 16 – Heart of Grateful

Bono, G., et al., "Gratitude in Practice and the Practice of Gratitude," in P.A. Linley and S. Joseph (Eds.), *Positive Psychology in Practice*, New York: Wiley

Childre, D., Martin, H., *The HeartMath Solution*, 1999, San Francisco: HarperCollins

Childre, D., *Overcoming Emotional Chaos*, 2003, San Diego, CA: Jodere Group

Emmons, R.A., McCullough, M.E., "Counting Blessings Versus Burdens: Experimental Studies of Gratitude and Subjective Well-Being," *Journal of Personality and Social Psychology*, 2003, 84:377-389

Emmons, R.A., McCullough, M.E. (Eds.), *The Psychology of Gratitude*, 2004, New York: Oxford University Press

Emmons, R.A., *Thanks! How the New Science of Gratitude Can Make You Happier*, 2007, New York: Houghton-Mifflin

Froh, J. J., Sefick, W. J., Emmons, R. A., "Counting Blessings in Early Adolescents: An Experimental Study of Gratitude and Subjective Well-being," *Journal of School Psychology*, 2008, 46(2):213-233

Goleman, D., *Emotional Intelligence: Why It Can Matter More Than IQ*, 2006, Bantam Books

McCullough, M. E., "Savoring Life, Past and Present: Explaining What Hope and Gratitude Share in Common," *Psychological Inquiry*, 2002, 13(4):302-304.

Seligman, M., *Authentic Happiness*, 2002, New York: The Free Press

Chapter 17 – Making a Difference

Benson, P.L., et al., "Altruism and Health: Is There a Link During Adolescence," *Altruism and Health: Perspectives from Empirical Research*, ed. Stephen G. Post, 2007, New York: Oxford University Press

Foresight, "Mental Capital and Wellbeing," Government Office for Science, United Kingdom, 2007

Krishna, R.M., M.D., "How Volunteerism Can Make You Happier and Healthier," *Integris (Online Journal)*

Kyrouz, E.M., et al., "A Review of Research on the Effectiveness of Self-Help Mutual Aid Groups," *American Self-Help Clearinghouse, Self-Help Group Sourcebook* (7th Edition)

Luks, A., (1988), "Doing Good: Helper's High," *Psychology Today*, 22(10)

Moll, J., et al., "Human Fronto-Mesolimbic Networks Guide Decisions About Charitable Donation," *Proceedings of the National Academy of Sciences of the United States of America*, 2006, 103(42)

Musick, M.A., Wilson, J., "Volunteering and Depression: The Role of Psychological and Social Resources in Different Age Groups," *Social Science & Medicine*, 2003, 56

Oman, D., et al., "Volunteerism and Mortality among the Community-Dwelling Elderly," *Journal of Health Psychology*, 1999, 4(3)

Post, S.G., "Altruism, Happiness, and Health: It's Good to Be Good," *International Journal of Behavioral Medicine*, 2005, 12(2)

Post, S., Neimark, J., *Why Good Things Happen to Good People*, 2007, New York: Broadway Books

Silverman, P., Ph.D., "Understanding Self-Help Groups," *The Self-Help Group Sourcebook: Your Guide to Community and Online Support Groups* (7th Edition), 2002, Denville, NJ: Saint Clare's Health Services

Speigel, D., *Living Beyond Limits*, 1994, Ballantine Books